# Pituitary Tumors

Lisa B. Nachtigall
Editor

# Pituitary Tumors

## A Clinical Casebook

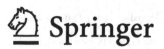
Springer

*Editor*
Lisa B. Nachtigall
Neuroendocrine Unit
Massachusetts General Hospital
Harvard Medical School
Boston, MA, USA

ISBN 978-3-319-90907-3 ISBN 978-3-319-90909-7 (eBook)
https://doi.org/10.1007/978-3-319-90909-7

Library of Congress Control Number: 2018949909

This Springer imprint is published by the registered company Springer Nature Switzerland AG
The registered company address is: Gewerbestrasse 11, 6330 Cham, Switzerland

*This book is dedicated to Dr. Anne Klibanski, who introduced me to pituitary tumors 25 years ago and from whom I continue to learn, and to Dr. Lila and Dr. Richard Nachtigall, who taught me the importance, of the patient as an individual and inspired my career in endocrinology.*

# Preface

*"Wherever the art of Medicine is loved, there is also a love of Humanity."*

—Hippocrates

Whether you are an expert on pituitary disorders, a student learning for the first time about this remarkable gland, or a physician or investigator who seeks a nuanced approach to the diagnosis and management of pituitary tumors, this casebook is for you. This is a collection of cases and their management, which aims to expand an understanding of pituitary tumors through the stories that unfold here of specific real life patient journeys, told by the clinician experts who cared for them.

The pituitary is a small pea-sized gland, but a powerful one which secretes hormones that control multiple endocrine axes: including the thyroid, reproductive, adrenal, and growth hormone axes. Hormone excess syndromes occur from functioning tumors which include acromegaly, gigantism, Cushing's disease, and prolactinomas. Hormone deficiencies can be caused by larger pituitary tumors, both functioning and nonfunctioning, that cause mass effect which may impair normal function of the anterior pituitary. All of these syndromes are described in case-based chapters, including at least one case of each type of tumor with a focus on the individual patient as an example of key points in diagnosis and management.

Many thanks to the authors who contributed chapters, as well as to the patients who shared their cases.

Boston, MA, USA                                                                    Lisa B. Nachtigall

# Contents

# Contributors

**Laura E. Dichtel, MD, MHS** Neuroendocrine Unit, Massachusetts General Hospital, Harvard Medical School, Boston, MA, USA

**Souad Enakuaa, MD** Neuroendocrine Unit, Massachusetts General Hospital, Harvard Medical School, Boston, MA, USA

**Pouneh K. Fazeli, MD, MPH** Neuroendocrine Unit, Massachusetts General Hospital, Harvard Medical School, Boston, MA, USA

**Lindsay Fourman, MD** Neuroendocrine Unit, Massachusetts General Hospital, Harvard Medical School, Boston, MA, USA

**Dariush Jahandideh, MD** Neuroendocrine Unit, Massachusetts General Hospital, Harvard Medical School, Boston, MA, USA

**Lisa B. Nachtigall, MD** Neuroendocrine Unit, Massachusetts General Hospital, Harvard Medical School, Boston, MA, USA

**Melanie Schorr, MD** Neuroendocrine Unit, Massachusetts General Hospital, Harvard Medical School, Boston, MA, USA

**Vibha Singhal, MD** Department of Pediatric Endocrinology, Massachusetts General Hospital, Harvard Medical School, Boston, MA, USA

**Suman Srinivasa, MD, MS** Neuroendocrine Unit, Massachusetts General Hospital, Harvard Medical School, Boston, MA, USA

**Nicholas A. Tritos, MD, DSc, FACP** Neuroendocrine Unit, Massachusetts General Hospital, Harvard Medical School, Boston, MA, USA

# Chapter 1
# Macroprolactinoma: Diagnosis and Management in a Patient with Infertility

Souad Enakuaa and Lisa B. Nachtigall

## Case Presentation

A 31-year-old female presented with secondary amenorrhea and infertility. Prior medical history was unremarkable except for delayed puberty. Her growth curve reportedly showed a low but constant height percentile. She had the onset of menarche at the age of 16 years. Her menstrual cycles had been consistently irregular since their onset, with periods every 1–3 months. She received oral contraceptives for a few years before discontinuing their use 1 year ago. She reported taking no medications upon her initial consultation with neuroendocrine.

On physical examination, her weight was 110 lb, height was 5 ft, blood pressure was 90/60, and heart rate was 64. The exam was notable for galactorrhea. Visual fields were normal. She had no evidence of Cushing's or acromegaly.

Initial hormonal analysis showed serum prolactin (diluted) level of 1048 ng/dL (normal range 5–20). FSH was 2.7 U/L, LH was 4.7 U/L, and estradiol level was low. Insulin-like growth fac-

S. Enakuaa · L. B. Nachtigall (✉)
Neuroendocrine Unit, Massachusetts General Hospital,
Harvard Medical School, Boston, MA, USA
e-mail: lnachtigall@partners.org

© Springer International Publishing AG, part of Springer Nature 2018
L. B. Nachtigall (ed.), *Pituitary Tumors*,
https://doi.org/10.1007/978-3-319-90909-7_1

tor 1 (IGF-1), free T4, and TSH were normal. HCG Quant was <6 IU/L. Her Cortrosyn stimulation test was normal with a stimulated peak cortisol level of 21.5 µg/dL (normal > 18). Pituitary magnetic resonance image (MRI) showed 1.4 cm macroadenoma without significant local invasion. Bone density was normal.

## My Management

- Initiated dopamine agonist therapy with cabergoline 0.5 mg orally weekly. After 3 months of cabergoline treatment, prolactin level was 23.2 ng/dL (0–20).
- Cabergoline dose was increased to 0.75 mg weekly. (The increase in dose was an effort to suppress tumor and also restore prolactin level to within the normal range, as to allow for return of menstrual cycle.)
- Three months later, progesterone level confirmed spontaneous ovulatory cycle.
- At 6 months follow-up, she reported the return of regular menstrual cycles while on 0.75 mg weekly of cabergoline with a prolactin level of 13 ng/dL, and MRI showed decrease in tumor size from 1.5 to 1 cm, with a question of an area of hemorrhage within the tumor.
- She was then referred to a neurosurgeon who suggested observation with close follow-up by MRI.
- After 10 months of cabergoline therapy (4 months after the prior MRI), her MRI was stable.
- After 18 months on cabergoline, she spontaneously conceived, and cabergoline was discontinued.
- She continued to follow up during pregnancy with observation of symptoms and exam including a neuro-ophthalmology exam with visual field testing every trimester.
- Three months postpartum prolactin level was 563 ng/dL. She opted to bottle-feed, but the amenorrhea persisted. Cabergoline was restarted and titrated to achieve a normal prolactin level and return of regular menstrual cycles.

## Assessment and Diagnosis

This patient presented with secondary amenorrhea and infertility, which are typical features of a prolactinoma. Primary amenorrhea and delayed puberty can be the initial presentation of this disease. Interestingly, she had delayed menarche and oligomenorrhea but had not undergone a pituitary evaluation until many years later when she presented with infertility. She is representative of cases in which the diagnosis of hyperprolactinemia is delayed and only discovered many years after a late puberty or late menarche [1]. Her late puberty may well have been due to hyperprolactinemia.

Detailed history of medications is important, as many commonly used drugs can cause hyperprolactinemia [2]. Metoclopramide, antipsychotics, antidepressants, antihypertensives, and opiates among many other pharmacological agents all may increase prolactin levels. Metoclopramide, haloperidol, risperidone, and phenothiazines may be associated with particularly elevated prolactin levels. Illicit drug use is another important history element because of the association of cocaine and heroin with hyperprolactinemia [3, 4].

Galactorrhea is present in less than half of patients with prolactinomas [5]. While in this case, her visual field exam was normal, it is important to evaluate visual field exams in any patient who has a lesion that extends to the suprasellar area and contacts or invades the optic chiasm.

There are many physiological causes of hyperprolactinemia including pregnancy, lactation, nipple stimulation, post-coitus state, and exercise. Pathological factors such as hypothyroidism, liver disease, renal failure, and seizure can also increase the prolactin level. Prolactinoma may co-secrete growth hormone. Therefore, IGF-1 should be evaluated to screen for acromegaly, particularly if there is clinical evidence of the disease. Typically prolactin levels greater than 250 ng/dL are associated with the presence of a prolactinoma [6]. A prolactin level above 500 ng/dL confirms prolactinoma as the diagnosis [7].

Our patient's initial level was above 1000 ng/dL, confirming the diagnosis of prolactinoma definitively. Pregnancy test and other hormonal assays of FSH, LH, TSH, and IGF-1 were normal. It is notable that rare cases of extremely high levels of prolactin can cause a false-negative assay result due to the "hook effect." In immunoassays, hook effect may occur when the amount of prolactin is so high that it impairs binding to antibody, causing falsely low results. To avoid the hook effect, the sample should be diluted with the patient's serum [8].

After confirming hyperprolactinemia and excluding other causes, imaging of the pituitary gland with an MRI is the next step. Prolactinomas are classified as either microprolactinoma (less than 1 cm) or a macroprolactinoma (greater than or equal to 1 cm). MRI is important for assessment of tumor size and to evaluate for mass effect on surrounding tissues. Ongoing imaging of the tumor is required in addition to biochemical testing to assess response to therapy. The presence of a macroadenoma on the MRI was expected in our patient given the severity of hyperprolactinemia, since an association between the degree of hyperprolactinemia and tumor size has been reported [9]. However, there are cases in which there can be discrepancy between the hormone levels and tumor size.

## Management

Once the diagnosis is established, goals of therapy should be set. In women, the goals are usually to restore menstrual cycle in reproductive age women and fertility in those who desire it. For women who are not trying to conceive, therapy should aim to avoid complications on bone health (which results from low estrogen levels, due to the suppression of gonadotropin-releasing hormone caused by hyperprolactinemia) [10] and to suppress tumor growth in order to prevent mass effects. Dopamine agonists (DAs) are the first line of therapy for prolactinomas [11]. DAs bind to dopamine receptors on lactotroph cells leading to decrease prolactin synthesis and reduction of tumor size [12, 13]. The currently available FDA-approved dopamine agonists in the USA that are used to treat hyperprolactinemia include bromocriptine and cabergoline. Both are effective in treating prolactinomas with a slight efficacy advantage of cabergoline [14, 15], which also has been associated with fewer side effects [15]. We typically suggest that the patients use or switch to bromocriptine prepregnancy since more data is available on its safety during pregnancy [5]. This patient preferred to stay on cabergoline since she tolerated it well and was concerned about having side effects if she switched drugs.

Surgery is another modality of treatment for macroprolactinoma. Surgical removal is not usually the first line of therapy but could be considered if there is optic chiasm compression affecting the visual field, bleeding within the tumor, or if the patient has a contraindication to use DAs, such as psychosis [16]. Surgery may also be appropriate if medical therapy fails and is not tolerable, if the tumor grows on medical therapy, or if a woman wants to conceive soon and has a large tumor [17]. Radiotherapy is reserved for prolactinomas that continue to grow after surgery, inoperable tumors, or patients who have failed to respond or tolerate medical therapy. Single-dose radiosurgery can be used in select cases of prolactinoma but is contraindicated if tumors are very large or approach the chiasm. In these cases, the risk of visual field loss is high with single-dose radiotherapy, and fractionated radiotherapy would be required [18].

## Outcome

The patient had a normal prolactin within 3 months of starting a low dose of cabergoline. This illustrated her dramatic response to this dopamine agonist with normalization of her prolactin level within a short period of time.

The return of spontaneous menstrual cycles occurred within weeks after she obtained a normal prolactin level, which is not uncommon [19], and was ultimately associated with spontaneous conception at 18 months after the initiation of dopamine agonist therapy. The time to obtaining fertility after correction of hyperprolactinemia is variable. Studies have shown that fertility can be restored within the first cycle after correction of high prolactin in some women but may take as long as 2 years [19] especially if there are other factors contributing to infertility. In this case, the patient's low weight when she first presented (BMI < 20) may have had a role in her infertility. It was after she had gained some weight that she ultimately conceived.

The patient developed the finding on MRI of a pre-contrast T1 bright spot, consistent with a possible area of hemorrhage, after the initiation of the dopamine agonist. While in this case, this was self-limited and follow-up imaging confirmed stability, a neurosurgical referral was obtained to entertain the possibility of surgical intervention if necessary.

Bleeding of the tumor is not an infrequent occurrence, especially in macroprolactinomas [20]. The bleeding can present as an emergency, as in the case of pituitary apoplexy. However, some degree of bleeding may be asymptomatic and resolves spontaneously [21]. Dopamine agonists are recognized as one of the precipitating factors of tumor hemorrhage and pituitary apoplexy [22]. Although this does not usually occur, most prolactinomas remain stable during pregnancy [23], but macroprolactinomas are more likely than microprolactinomas to grow during gestation [23]. Safety of DAs during pregnancy is not completely known, and thus both cabergoline and bromocriptine are class B medications, as designated by the FDA. However, observational data of fetal exposure either in the first trimester or throughout pregnancy to both bromocriptine and cabergoline did not show any significant harm [5]. Recommended management is stopping the dopamine agonist as soon as the pregnancy is known. Follow-up of the tumor size should be performed by relevant symptom review and visual field examination in every trimester. Prolactin level is not meaningful during pregnancy because hyperprolactinemia is physiological and expected during pregnancy. If there is any change in the symptoms suggestive of tumor enlargement, official visual field evaluation and non-contrast MRI should be obtained. Our patient had normal visual fields throughout her pregnancy. Postpartum her prolactin levels remained elevated despite the fact that she was not nursing and her menstrual periods did not resume. For that reason, the cabergoline was restarted postpartum and again associated with return of regular cycles and normalization of prolactin, and she had ongoing improvement with decrease in pituitary tumor size.

### Clinical Pearls and Pitfalls
- Delayed puberty may be a sign of hyperprolactinemia.
- Prolactin level should be evaluated in women with absent or irregular menses prior to initiating birth control pills.
- When prolactin level is very high, diluted prolactin should be obtained to avoid the hook effect if an immunoassay is used.
- Even though her prolactin level normalized within 3 months of therapy with a dopamine agonist, her persistence of a

macroadenoma remained. This illustrates the importance of following both the biochemical parameters and the imaging in patients with macroprolactinomas who were treated medically.

- While the prolactin trend will typically mirror the tumor size response, they are not always completely linked [24].
- One of the consequences of a dopamine agonist in patients with a prolactinoma can include hemorrhage into the tumor. This requires close follow-up with imaging and neurosurgical consultation as well as evaluation of anterior pituitary function, particularly if symptoms of apoplexy are present.
- Lactotroph hyperplasia can occur during normal pregnancy, and in patients with macroprolactinoma, enlargement during pregnancy is a concern, as the risk of growth is much greater than that of microprolactinoma [23]. Therefore, visual field tests were done each trimester and are important in the management of patients with macroprolactinomas during pregnancy.

# References

1. Landolt AM. [Prolactin-producing pituitary adenomas as a cause of primary amenorrhea and their neurosurgical treatment]. Dtsch Med Wochenschr. 1983;108(8):298–301.
2. Ajmal A, Joffe H, Nachtigall LB. Psychotropic-induced hyperprolactinemia: a clinical review. Psychosomatics. 2014;55(1):29–36.
3. Shin SH, et al. Morphine can stimulate prolactin release independent of a dopaminergic mechanism. Can J Physiol Pharmacol. 1988;66(11):1381–5.
4. Gold MS, et al. Increase in serum prolactin by exogenous and endogenous opiates: evidence for antidopamine and antipsychotic effects. Am J Psychiatry. 1978;135(11):1415–6.
5. Glezer A, Bronstein MD. Prolactinomas, cabergoline, and pregnancy. Endocrine. 2014;47(1):64–9.
6. Melmed S, et al. Diagnosis and treatment of hyperprolactinemia: an Endocrine Society clinical practice guideline. J Clin Endocrinol Metab. 2011;96(2):273–88.
7. Vilar L, Fleseriu M, Bronstein MD. Challenges and pitfalls in the diagnosis of hyperprolactinemia. Arq Bras Endocrinol Metabol. 2014;58(1):9–22.

8. St-Jean E, Blain F, Comtois R. High prolactin levels may be missed by immunoradiometric assay in patients with macroprolactinomas. Clin Endocrinol (Oxf). 1996;44(3):305–9.
9. Moraes AB, et al. Giant prolactinomas: the therapeutic approach. Clin Endocrinol (Oxf). 2013;79(4):447–56.
10. Brue T, Castinetti F. The risks of overlooking the diagnosis of secreting pituitary adenomas. Orphanet J Rare Dis. 2016;11(1):135.
11. Faje A, Nachtigall L. Current treatment options for hyperprolactinemia. Expert Opin Pharmacother. 2013;14(12):1611–25.
12. Biller BM, et al. Treatment of prolactin-secreting macroadenomas with the once-weekly dopamine agonist cabergoline. J Clin Endocrinol Metab. 1996;81(6):2338–43.
13. Molitch ME, et al. Bromocriptine as primary therapy for prolactin-secreting macroadenomas: results of a prospective multicenter study. J Clin Endocrinol Metab. 1985;60(4):698–705.
14. Colao A, et al. Long-term and low-dose treatment with cabergoline induces macroprolactinoma shrinkage. J Clin Endocrinol Metab. 1997;82(11):3574–9.
15. Webster J, et al. A comparison of cabergoline and bromocriptine in the treatment of hyperprolactinemic amenorrhea. Cabergoline Comparative Study Group. N Engl J Med. 1994;331(14):904–9.
16. Donegan D, et al. Surgical outcomes of prolactinomas in recent era: results of a heterogenous group. Endocr Pract. 2017;23(1):37–45.
17. Wilson CB. Surgical management of pituitary tumors. J Clin Endocrinol Metab. 1997;82(8):2381–5.
18. Pashtan I, Oh KS, Loeffler JS. Radiation therapy in the management of pituitary adenomas. Handb Clin Neurol. 2014;124:317–24.
19. Ono M, et al. Individualized high-dose cabergoline therapy for hyperprolactinemic infertility in women with micro- and macroprolactinomas. J Clin Endocrinol Metab. 2010;95(6):2672–9.
20. Sarwar KN, et al. The prevalence and natural history of pituitary hemorrhage in prolactinoma. J Clin Endocrinol Metab. 2013;98(6):2362–7.
21. Watt A, Pobereskin L, Vaidya B. Pituitary apoplexy within a macroprolactinoma. Nat Clin Pract Endocrinol Metab. 2008;4(11):635–41.
22. Briet C, et al. Pituitary apoplexy. Endocr Rev. 2015;36(6):622–45.
23. Molitch ME. Endocrinology in pregnancy: management of the pregnant patient with a prolactinoma. Eur J Endocrinol. 2015;172(5):R205–13.
24. Maiter D, Delgrange E. Therapy of endocrine disease: the challenges in managing giant prolactinomas. Eur J Endocrinol. 2014;170(6):R213–27.

# Chapter 2
# Macroprolactinoma: Alternatives to Dopamine Agonist Therapy for Treatment of Macroprolactinomas in Patients Who Present with Psychotic Symptoms

Suman Srinivasa

## Case Presentation

This is a 22-year-old male with no significant past medical history who presented with progressive vision loss for 3 months. Formal visual field testing was obtained through the patient's ophthalmologist, which demonstrated a bitemporal hemianopsia. A pituitary MRI was ordered, which revealed a sellar and suprasellar mass measuring 42 × 30 × 38 mm in size with compression of the optic chiasm and invasion of the right cavernous sinus. The patient denied any complaints of headache. Biochemical testing was significant for elevated prolactin of 4064 ng/mL and a low free T4 (FT4) of 0.8 ng/dL. The patient was exonerated of adrenal insufficiency through cosyntropin stimulation testing. The remainder of his pituitary function was unremarkable, and there was no evidence of cosecretion. The patient was started on cabergoline 0.5 mg daily for a presumed macroprolactinoma. A relatively

S. Srinivasa (✉)
Neuroendocrine Unit, Massachusetts General Hospital,
Harvard Medical School, Boston, MA, USA
e-mail: ssrinivasa@mgh.harvard.edu

© Springer International Publishing AG, part of Springer Nature 2018
L. B. Nachtigall (ed.), *Pituitary Tumors*,
https://doi.org/10.1007/978-3-319-90909-7_2

higher dose was initiated given the urgency to preserve visual function. A prolactin and pituitary MRI were reevaluated after 2 weeks. The prolactin level was significantly reduced to 657 ng/mL. Repeat MRI showed a decrease in size of the macroprolactinoma now measuring 30 × 27 × 33 mm in size with decompression of the optic chiasm. The patient's cabergoline dose was reduced to 0.5 mg twice weekly, as the proximity of the tumor to the optic chiasm became less concerning. He continued to demonstrate a good biochemical and tumor response. After 1 month of medical therapy, the prolactin level was 25 ng/mL. Normalization of the prolactin was later achieved by 8 months, but imaging of the pituitary was notable for stable residual tumor. Two years following a stable dose of cabergoline, the patient reported new-onset auditory hallucinations, delusions, and excessive anxiety, which profoundly impaired his social and professional interactions.

## My Management Options

(a) Start antipsychotic medications, and continue to treat the macroprolactinoma with cabergoline.
(b) Discontinue the cabergoline and refer to neurosurgery to remove the residual tumor.
(c) Discontinue the cabergoline and refer to radiation oncology for radiation therapy.

## Assessment and Diagnosis

Prolactin is regulated primarily through dopamine via negative feedback. Dopamine is secreted from neurons of the arcuate nucleus in the tuberoinfundibular pathway and has an inhibitory effect on prolactin synthesis and secretion by binding to dopamine D2 receptors found on lactotrophs in the anterior pituitary gland [1]. In contrast, thyrotropin-releasing hormone has a smaller contribution to regulating prolactin through stimulation of prolactin release [2].

Based on this physiology, dopamine agonists are the treatment of choice to reduce prolactin levels and lactotroph hyperplasia. Cabergoline is an ergot derivative which demonstrates good efficacy for treatment of prolactinomas due to its high binding affinity for dopamine D2 receptors. Cabergoline is often preferred to bromocriptine for managing prolactinomas due to superior efficacy [3] probably due to greater selectivity for the dopamine D2 receptor, longer half-life, and better tolerated side effects, such as nausea and orthostasis.

An additional concern with the use of dopamine agonists for prolactinomas is the development of psychotic symptoms [4]. Based on the elimination half-life of cabergoline, systemic levels of the medication may be present for a few weeks. A single dose of cabergoline can have lasting effects on the prolactin for 21 days [5]. Cases of psychosis have been reported with use of cabergoline and bromocriptine for treatment of prolactinomas [6, 7]. Some reports have suggested that psychotic symptoms decrease after withdrawal of the dopamine agonist. Currently, there are no data to suggest differential effects on the severity of psychotic symptoms between cabergoline and bromocriptine based on varying pharmacokinetic profiles, and both medications should be used with caution, in consultation with psychiatry, or avoided, if psychosis is suspected.

A clear dose-dependent relationship between cabergoline use and psychotic symptoms remains unknown. Higher doses of cabergoline are used to treat Parkinson's disease, and cases of psychosis are similarly reported in these patients [8]. Regardless of the dose, symptoms of psychosis need to be monitored cautiously. Lowering the dose of cabergoline may be a plausible strategy. However, cases of psychosis have been reported on low doses of dopamine agonists [9], and there are no safety data related to psychosis to support this management and is not generally advised. In addition, there are reports of persistent psychiatric decompensation despite the addition of an antipsychotic drug to a dopamine agonist, and therefore, concomitant use of the two agents is not typically recommended for management of a prolactinoma as well [10, 11]. The risks of psychiatric decompensation may outweigh the potential risks of a prolactinoma, as there are alternative approaches for safely managing prolactinomas.

While there is no clear mechanism for psychosis, dopamine hypersensitivity is hypothesized to play a key role. In this regard, dopamine antagonists are commonly used to treat antipsychotic disorders and demonstrate efficacy in psychosis by blocking the dopamine receptors in the mesolimbic pathway. Common symptoms of psychotic disorders include delusions and hallucinations as well as loss of emotion, speech, or motivation. Through their mechanism of action to block dopamine D2 receptors, dopamine antagonist use can result in unwanted side effects, such as medication-induced hyperprolactinemia by blocking the tonic inhibition of prolactin, thereby leading to increased prolactin levels. In addition, other classes of psychiatric medications, such as SSRIs, may also have unintended consequences of hyperprolactinemia [12].

While in this scenario, cabergoline was initiated first to treat a macroprolactinoma, prior reports exploring the commencement of cabergoline following antipsychotic therapy for medication-induced hyperprolactinemia are important to understand the interaction between these two classes of medications. Some reports had suggested that dopamine agonists, such as cabergoline, could be safely administered to treat medication-induced hyperprolactinemia secondary to antipsychotic use [13, 14]. However, in light of new evidence to suggest that dopamine agonists have the potential to exacerbate psychosis, this management is not recommended. While limited data are available evaluating the causal relationship between cabergoline and psychiatric disease, case reports suggest a significant and worrisome association is present [15–17]. Moreover, additional links of dopamine agonists to heightened impulsivity [18, 19] and mania [17, 20] in patients treated for prolactinomas have also been described in the literature.

## Management

Surgical intervention with a transsphenoidal resection even performed by the most experienced neurosurgeon is less likely to result in long-term biochemical remission and control of tumor growth [21–25] when compared to medical therapy for prolactin-secreting tumors. Therefore, first-line treatment for a macroprolactinoma is dopamine agonist therapy. Alternatives to medical therapy may be warranted under special clinical circumstances, such as intolerance to dopamine agonist therapy, absolute or relative contraindication to dopamine agonist therapy, or poor response (either by biochemical or tumor measures) to dopamine agonist therapy. In this case, this patient was considered to have a contraindication to dopamine agonists based on the exacerbation of his psychosis. While surgical management could be offered as the next step, there were other considerations unique to this case, such as the patient's age and aggressive nature of the tumor. The early onset of his disease presentation and characteristics of tumor aggressiveness (cavernous sinus invasion) increase the probability for potential recurrence that may require additional long-term treatment.

More definitive treatment with radiation should be considered when disease chronicity or aggressive features are a concern. Long-term consequences of radiation therapy should be discussed with the patient, the most common of which is hypopituitarism. The development of a secondary malignancy or neurologic symptoms, such as optic neuropathy and stroke are less common. Hypopituitarism can be managed with hormone replacement, and the usual onset does not occur on average until many years from treatment [26].

As approximately 90% of prolactinomas respond to dopamine agonist therapy, few cases require use of surgery or radiation. In this regard, data on the efficacy of transsphenoidal resection and radiation therapy is limited. One retrospective study following surgical intervention for prolactinoma reported an initial remission rate of 53%, which later declined to 43%, and the overall recurrence rate was 19% [27]. Other prospective studies demonstrate similar recurrence rates [21]. Data also show that prolactin-secreting macroadenomas and invasive adenomas tend to have reduced rates of remission and complete eradication of tumor [22, 28] when compared to microprolactinomas. Certainly, surgical intervention may be an option in situations where debulking is necessary or to facilitate adjunctive radiation [29]. In a series of 128 patients followed after receiving gamma knife radiation, 67 cases achieved clinical cure. Most patients demonstrated tumor control, but about 1/3 of patients followed for over 2 years still had evidence of hyperprolactinemia [30]. Another center's experience with radiation similarly showed good tumor control and less frequent biochemical control among prolactinomas treated with radiation and followed up to a median of 6 years [31]. More recent data on proton therapy demonstrated that about 98% of all adenomas respond to treatment; however, two of three patients that had radiographic progression were prolactin-secreting adenomas. Biochemical remission was achieved in 38% of the prolactinoma cases by 5 years, a rate much lower than the other subtypes of adenomas [32]. Overall, response to radiation for prolactinomas tends to be less frequent and delayed when compared to other adenomas.

In addition, treatment of the underlying psychiatric disease should be pursued in consultation with the psychiatrist. Elevated prolactin levels are present in over 70% of patients on risperidone [33, 34] and may be elevated to a lesser extent in other atypical antipsychotics, such as olanzapine and clozapine. As clozapine has a weak binding affinity to the dopamine D2 receptor, hyperprolactinemia is rare [35], but its use may be limited by considerable side effects. Using an antipsychotic agent which tends to have fewer effects on the prolactin may be preferred, but ultimately the patient should be treated as necessary to stabilize the psychosis.

Aripiprazole is an ideal choice to dually manage psychosis and hyperprolactinemia if tolerated by the patient [34, 36] and administered in consultation with the managing psychiatrist. Aripiprazole's mechanism of action as a partial dopamine agonist gives it the advantage to treat psychotic symptoms while lowering prolactin levels [37, 38]. Further investigation into aripiprazole's effect on tumor size is needed, but isolated case reports suggest a beneficial reduction in prolactinoma size [39].

## Outcome

Indeed, this case demonstrates the initial efficacy of cabergoline, as there was a rapid response in the prolactin level and tumor size. The patient's clinical course was interrupted by serious psychiatric complaints, which prompted the immediate discontinuation of cabergoline. He was referred to psychiatry and was newly diagnosed with psychosis. The exacerbation of his psychotic symptoms had a significant impact on his life, leading to social isolation and a temporary leave of absence from his career. Upon further questioning, the patient expressed that mild anxiety and paranoia existed in the years prior to diagnosis of his macroprolactinoma. He was able to manage his symptoms conservatively through coping strategies and, therefore, never brought these symptoms to the attention of his care providers, as may be a common scenario in high-functioning individuals.

Following discontinuation of the cabergoline, the prolactin level rose to 838 ng/dL. In addition, the prolactin rose further to 992 ng/dL after olanzapine, an atypical antipsychotic and dopamine antagonist, was initiated to treat his auditory hallucinations and delusions. Aripiprazole was considered to manage the psychotic symptoms, but he did not tolerate this well. Olanzapine was continued to provide optimal psychiatric benefit. He was simultaneously referred to radiation oncology for further management of the macroprolactinoma.

The patient was advised to undergo fractionated radiation, which was tolerated well. Pituitary MRI at 6-, 12-, and 24-months postradiation demonstrated stability of the tumor. Two years following radiation, the prolactin level had decreased by half to 428 ng/dL, while the patient actively remained on a dopamine antagonist for his psychiatric illness. Overall, his social and professional impairment had been slowly improving with titration of his dopamine antagonist treatment.

The patient subsequently developed fatigue and decreased libido. A morning testosterone level was 19 ng/dL, which was consistent with male hypogonadism. The hypogonadism probably developed after prolactin levels rose due to withdrawal of cabergoline therapy. In males, hypogonadism may be the initial presenting symptoms in cases of hyperprolactinemia [40]. Hyperprolactinemia contributes to hypogonadism through suppressive effects on gonadotrophin-releasing hormone. Testosterone replacement was started. A normal testosterone level was achieved (336 ng/dL) despite ongoing biochemical evidence of hyperprolactinemia, and symptoms related to hypogonadism eventually resolved.

**Clinical Pearls and Pitfalls**

- Prior to starting a dopamine agonist, physicians should screen patients for psychiatric disease. When a psychiatric disorder is suspected, referral to a psychiatrist is recommended to determine if starting a dopamine agonist is clinically feasible. Use of a dopamine agonist is not recommended in psychotic patients and may have detrimental effects on social and professional functioning.

- Dopamine agonists can unmask an underlying psychotic disorder. If an unknown psychiatric condition is exacerbated after starting a dopamine agonist, the medication should be discontinued.

- Antipsychotic agents functioning as dopamine antagonists may contribute to medication-induced hyperprolactinemia. Any underlying psychiatric disorder should be treated as deemed appropriate by the psychiatrist. The preferred antipsychotic to treat symptoms of psychosis in the setting of hyperprolactinemia is aripiprazole [41], which functions as a partial dopamine agonist and may reduce prolactin levels. Data are lacking as to aripiprazole's effects on tumor growth.

- Surgery and/or radiation therapy can be effective second-line treatment strategies for macroprolactinomas not amenable to medical therapy. When there is residual tissue or aggressive features, transsphenoidal resection may not be entirely effective but can be considered for debulking, and radiation, either single dose or fractionated, may be the preferred option.

- In the setting of continued hyperprolactinemia following radiation, conservative monitoring is sufficient if the patient does not demonstrate any prolactin-related symptoms, as it is expected that tumor growth will stabilize and prolactin levels will gradually decline with radiation therapy.

- If patients cannot tolerate dopamine agonists, secondary symptoms should be treated via alternative methods. For example, male hypogonadism secondary to hyperprolactinemia can be alternatively treated with testosterone replacement, rather than with cabergoline. Female hypogonadism may require oral contraceptive therapy. Longstanding hypogonadism may have deleterious effects on quality of life and bone health and should be addressed [42, 43].

# References

1. Leblanc H, Lachelin GC, Abu-Fadil S, Yen SS. Effects of dopamine infusion on pituitary hormone secretion in humans. J Clin Endocrinol Metab. 1976;43:668–74.
2. Jacobs LS, Snyder PJ, Wilber JF, Utiger RD, Daughaday WH. Increased serum prolactin after administration of synthetic thyrotropin releasing hormone (TRH) in man. J Clin Endocrinol Metab. 1971;33:996–8.
3. Biller BM, Molitch ME, Vance ML, Cannistraro KB, Davis KR, Simons JA, Schoenfelder JR, Klibanski A. Treatment of prolactin-secreting macroadenomas with the once-weekly dopamine agonist cabergoline. J Clin Endocrinol Metab. 1996;81:2338–43.
4. Ali S, Miller KK, Freudenreich O. Management of psychosis associated with a prolactinoma: case report and review of the literature. Psychosomatics. 2010;51:370–6.
5. DA agonists—ergot derivatives: cabergoline: management of Parkinson's disease. Mov Disord. 2002;17 Suppl 4:S68–71.
6. Cabeza GA, Flores LF, Iniguez IE, Calarco ZE, Valencia PF. Acute psychosis secondary to bromocriptine treatment in a patient with a prolactinoma. Rev Invest Clin. 1984;36:147–9.
7. Peter SA, Autz A, Jean-Simon ML. Bromocriptine-induced schizophrenia. J Natl Med Assoc. 1993;85:700–1.
8. Weintraub D, Siderowf AD, Potenza MN, Goveas J, Morales KH, Duda JE, Moberg PJ, Stern MB. Association of dopamine agonist use with impulse control disorders in Parkinson disease. Arch Neurol. 2006;63:969–73.
9. Turner TH, Cookson JC, Wass JA, Drury PL, Price PA, Besser GM. Psychotic reactions during treatment of pituitary tumours with dopamine agonists. Br Med J (Clin Res Ed). 1984;289:1101–3.
10. Nieman DH, Sutterland AL, Otten J, Becker HE, Drent ML, van der Gaag M, Birchwood M, de Haan L. Treating prolactinoma and psychosis: medication and cognitive behavioural therapy. BMJ Case Rep. 2011;1–5.
11. Robbins RJ, Kern PA, Thompson TL 2nd. Interactions between thioridazine and bromocriptine in a patient with a prolactin-secreting pituitary adenoma. Am J Med. 1984;76:921–3.

12. Papakostas GI, Miller KK, Petersen T, Sklarsky KG, Hilliker SE, Klibanski A, Fava M. Serum prolactin levels among outpatients with major depressive disorder during the acute phase of treatment with fluoxetine. J Clin Psychiatry. 2006;67:952–7.

13. Tollin SR. Use of the dopamine agonists bromocriptine and cabergoline in the management of risperidone-induced hyperprolactinemia in patients with psychotic disorders. J Endocrinol Invest. 2000;23:765–70.

14. Cavallaro R, Cocchi F, Angelone SM, Lattuada E, Smeraldi E. Cabergoline treatment of risperidone-induced hyperprolactinemia: a pilot study. J Clin Psychiatry. 2004;65:187–90.

15. Bilal L, Ching C. Cabergoline-induced psychosis in a patient with undiagnosed depression. J Neuropsychiatry Clin Neurosci. 2012;24:E54.

16. Chang SC, Chen CH, Lu ML. Cabergoline-induced psychotic exacerbation in schizophrenic patients. Gen Hosp Psychiatry. 2008;30:378–80.

17. Harris YT, Harris AZ, Deasis JM, Ferrando SJ, Reddy N, Young RC. Cabergoline associated with first episode mania. Psychosomatics. 2012;53:595–600.

18. Barake M, Evins AE, Stoeckel L, Pachas GN, Nachtigall LB, Miller KK, Biller BM, Tritos NA, Klibanski A. Investigation of impulsivity in patients on dopamine agonist therapy for hyperprolactinemia: a pilot study. Pituitary. 2014;17:150–6.

19. Martinkova J, Trejbalova L, Sasikova M, Benetin J, Valkovic P. Impulse control disorders associated with dopaminergic medication in patients with pituitary adenomas. Clin Neuropharmacol. 2011;34:179–81.

20. Yuksel RN, Elyas Kaya Z, Dilbaz N, Cingi Yirun M. Cabergoline-induced manic episode: case report. Ther Adv Psychopharmacol. 2016;6:229–31.

21. Feigenbaum SL, Downey DE, Wilson CB, Jaffe RB. Transsphenoidal pituitary resection for preoperative diagnosis of prolactin-secreting pituitary adenoma in women: long term follow-up. J Clin Endocrinol Metab. 1996;81:1711–9.

22. Randall RV, Laws ER Jr, Abboud CF, Ebersold MJ, Kao PC, Scheithauer BW. Transsphenoidal microsurgical treatment of prolactin-producing pituitary adenomas. Results in 100 patients. Mayo Clin Proc. 1983;58:108–21.

23. Schlechte JA, Sherman BM, Chapler FK, VanGilder J. Long term follow-up of women with surgically treated prolactin-secreting pituitary tumors. J Clin Endocrinol Metab. 1986;62:1296–301.

24. Serri O, Rasio E, Beauregard H, Hardy J, Somma M. Recurrence of hyperprolactinemia after selective transsphenoidal adenomectomy in women with prolactinoma. N Engl J Med. 1983;309:280–3.

25. Kristof RA, Schramm J, Redel L, Neuloh G, Wichers M, Klingmuller D. Endocrinological outcome following first time transsphenoidal surgery for GH-, ACTH-, and PRL-secreting pituitary adenomas. Acta Neurochir (Wien). 2002;144:555–561; discussion 561.

26. Snyder PJ, Fowble BF, Schatz NJ, Savino PJ, Gennarelli TA. Hypopituitarism following radiation therapy of pituitary adenomas. Am J Med. 1986;81:457–62.

27. Kreutzer J, Buslei R, Wallaschofski H, Hofmann B, Nimsky C, Fahlbusch R, Buchfelder M. Operative treatment of prolactinomas: indications and results in a current consecutive series of 212 patients. Eur J Endocrinol. 2008;158:11–8.

28. Primeau V, Raftopoulos C, Maiter D. Outcomes of transsphenoidal surgery in prolactinomas: improvement of hormonal control in dopamine agonist-resistant patients. Eur J Endocrinol. 2012;166:779–86.

29. Shimon I, Sosa E, Mendoza V, Greenman Y, Tirosh A, Espinosa E, Popovic V, Glezer A, Bronstein MD, Mercado M. Giant prolactinomas larger than 60 mm in size: a cohort of massive and aggressive prolactin-secreting pituitary adenomas. Pituitary. 2016;19:429–36.

30. Pan L, Zhang N, Wang EM, Wang BJ, Dai JZ, Cai PW. Gamma knife radiosurgery as a primary treatment for prolactinomas. J Neurosurg. 2000;93(Suppl 3):10–3.

31. Wilson PJ, Williams JR, Smee RI. Single-centre experience of stereotactic radiosurgery and fractionated stereotactic radiotherapy for prolactinomas with the linear accelerator. J Med Imaging Radiat Oncol. 2015;59:371–8.

32. Wattson DA, Tanguturi SK, Spiegel DY, Niemierko A, Biller BM, Nachtigall LB, Bussiere MR, Swearingen B, Chapman PH, Loeffler JS, Shih HA. Outcomes of proton therapy for patients with functional pituitary adenomas. Int J Radiat Oncol Biol Phys. 2014;90:532–9.

33. Molitch ME. Medication-induced hyperprolactinemia. Mayo Clin Proc. 2005;80:1050–7.

34. Potkin SG, Saha AR, Kujawa MJ, Carson WH, Ali M, Stock E, Stringfellow J, Ingenito G, Marder SR. Aripiprazole, an antipsychotic with a novel mechanism of action, and risperidone vs placebo in patients with schizophrenia and schizoaffective disorder. Arch Gen Psychiatry. 2003;60:681–90.

35. Volavka J, Czobor P, Cooper TB, Sheitman B, Lindenmayer JP, Citrome L, McEvoy JP, Lieberman JA. Prolactin levels in schizophrenia and schizoaffective disorder patients treated with clozapine, olanzapine, risperidone, or haloperidol. J Clin Psychiatry. 2004;65:57–61.

36. Hoffer ZS, Roth RL, Mathews M. Evidence for the partial dopamine-receptor agonist aripiprazole as a first-line treatment of psychosis in patients with iatrogenic or tumorogenic hyperprolactinemia. Psychosomatics. 2009;50:317–24.

37. Byerly M, Suppes T, Tran QV, Baker RA. Clinical implications of anti-psychotic-induced hyperprolactinemia in patients with schizophrenia spectrum or bipolar spectrum disorders: recent developments and current perspectives. J Clin Psychopharmacol. 2007;27:639–61.

38. Sheldrick AJ, Grunder G. Aripiprazole reduces serum prolactin in a woman with prolactinoma and acute psychosis. Pharmacopsychiatry. 2008;41:160.

39. Bakker IC, Schubart CD, Zelissen PM. Successful treatment of a prolactinoma with the antipsychotic drug aripiprazole. Endocrinol Diabetes Metab Case Rep. 2016;2016:160028.

40. Tsigkaropoulou E, Peppa M, Zompola C, Rizos E, Xelioti I, Chatziioannou S, Filippopoulou A, Lykouras L. Hypogonadism due to hyperprolactinemia and subsequent first episode of psychosis. Gend Med. 2012;9:56–60.
41. Wix-Ramos RJ, Paez R, Capote E, Ezequiel U. Pituitary microadenoma treated with antipsychotic drug aripiprazole. Recent Pat Endocr Metab Immune Drug Discov. 2011;5:58–60.
42. Klibanski A, Neer RM, Beitins IZ, Ridgway EC, Zervas NT, McArthur JW. Decreased bone density in hyperprolactinemic women. N Engl J Med. 1980;303:1511–4.
43. Greenspan SL, Neer RM, Ridgway EC, Klibanski A. Osteoporosis in men with hyperprolactinemic hypogonadism. Ann Intern Med. 1986;104:777–82.

# Chapter 3
# Nonfunctioning Pituitary Adenoma: Management

Melanie Schorr

## Case Presentation

A 65-year-old man was referred to the neuroendocrine clinic after failing a cosyntropin stimulation test and being diagnosed with central adrenal insufficiency during a hospital admission for fatigue and hypotension. Pituitary MRI during that admission demonstrated a 10 mm sellar lesion approaching, but not impinging, on the optic chiasm. His review of symptoms was otherwise negative, including no headaches, vision changes, low libido, erectile dysfunction, or galactorrhea. His other anterior pituitary hormones included serum TSH 0.54 uIU/mL (0.35–5.5), Free T4 (fT4) 1.29 ng/dL (0.8–1.9), 8 AM total testosterone 258 ng/dL, IGF-1 66 ng/mL (20–176), and prolactin 9.8 ng/mL (0–15). His medications included prednisone 5 mg QAM for adrenal insufficiency and levothyroxine 100 mcg QAM for a prior diagnosis of primary hypothyroidism. He was referred to a neuro-ophthalmologist, and visual field and visual acuity testing was normal. Repeat pituitary MRI in 6 months demonstrated that the mass had increased in size to 12 mm in the largest dimension, but was not impinging on the optic chiasm. Pituitary hormone testing, as well as visual field and visual acuity testing, at that time was stable. Pituitary MRI another 6 months thereafter demonstrated that the

M. Schorr (✉)
Neuroendocrine Unit, Massachusetts General Hospital,
Harvard Medical School, Boston, MA, USA
e-mail: mschorr1@partners.org

© Springer International Publishing AG, part of Springer Nature 2018　　21
L. B. Nachtigall (ed.), *Pituitary Tumors*,
https://doi.org/10.1007/978-3-319-90909-7_3

sellar lesion was now 14 mm in the largest dimension and close to impinging on the optic chiasm. Pituitary hormone testing, as well as visual field and visual acuity testing, was again stable.

## My Management

1. Observe for tumor growth with serial MRI's.
2. Refer to neurosurgeon for transsphenoidal surgery.
3. Initiate therapy with stress dose steroids perioperatively, given adrenal insufficiency.
4. Postoperative monitoring of sodium and anterior pituitary function.

## Assessment and Diagnosis

Pituitary adenomas are characterized by their size (microadenomas < 1 cm, macroadenomas ≥ 1 cm) and cell of origin (lactotroph, somatotroph, corticotroph, gonadotroph, and thyrotroph). Most adenomas (approximately 70%) are functioning tumors that secrete an excess amount of hormone and cause a clinical syndrome [1]. The remaining 30% of pituitary adenomas are considered clinically nonfunctioning, although 80–90% do produce intact gonadotropins or their subunits. However, clinical syndromes due to excess gonadotropin secretion are rare because gonadotroph adenomas are usually poorly differentiated and rarely cause elevated sex steroid levels [2].

Since nonfunctioning pituitary adenomas do not present with a clinical syndrome of pituitary hormone excess, the presentation may instead include the following:

1. Neurologic symptoms, such as visual impairment and/or headache. Most commonly this is visual field loss due to the adenoma's suprasellar extension resulting in optic chiasm compression and bitemporal hemianopsia. When the optic chiasm is severely compressed, decreased visual acuity may occur. Compression of the oculomotor nerve due to cavernous sinus invasion of the adenoma may result in diplopia. Headaches are a less common

presentation, but a new excruciating headache with new visual impairment must raise concern for pituitary apoplexy, which may be life-threatening due to acute secondary adrenal insufficiency [3].

2. Pituitary hormone deficiency due to mass effect from the adenoma. Symptoms of pituitary hormone deficiency are often nonspecific and may therefore go undiagnosed for some time. In a series of patients with nonfunctioning pituitary adenomas, 37–85% of patients had laboratory evidence of at least one pituitary hormone deficiency [4, 5], whereas panhypopituitarism was noted in 6–29% of patients [6, 7].

3. An incidental sellar mass on an imaging study not performed for pituitary disease. Given the prevalence of pituitary adenomas on autopsy series (10.6%), this is not an uncommon presentation of a nonfunctioning pituitary adenoma [8].

In accordance with the Endocrine Society Clinical Practice Guidelines on Pituitary Incidentalomas, the evaluation of a newly diagnosed sellar mass >1 cm in size should include a detailed history and physical exam, a dedicated pituitary MRI, biochemical evaluation of pituitary hormone excess and deficiency, and visual field and visual acuity testing if clinically indicated [9]. Visual testing may not be required if the pituitary MRI clearly shows no evidence of optic chiasm or cranial nerve involvement, the patient has no new visual symptoms, and the patient is being followed closely by MRI. Although pituitary adenomas are the most common cause of a sellar mass >1 cm, the differential diagnosis is large and includes craniopharyngioma, meningioma, metastatic tumors, Rathke's cleft cyst, and hypophysitis, which is why a thorough evaluation is prudent [10]. Biochemical evaluation for pituitary hormone excess may include serum prolactin, insulin-like growth factor 1 (IGF-1), TSH and FT4, and 24 hour (24-h) urine free cortisol and/or late-night salivary cortisol. Hyperprolactinemia may be consequent to pituitary stalk compression by a sellar mass or due to a pituitary lactotroph adenoma. Hyperprolactinemia secondary to stalk compression is due to obstruction of normal hypothalamic dopamine inhibition on pituitary lactotroph cells and typically results in serum prolactin levels <100 ng/mL, which can be used as a cutoff to help distinguish between a nonfunctioning pituitary macroadenoma with stalk compression and a pituitary lactotroph macroadenoma, the latter of which typically has serum prolactin levels >100 ng/mL [11]. In patients with pituitary macroadenomas, the laboratory should measure serum prolactin levels in dilution to ensure that levels are not falsely lowered by a hook effect in the assay. Biochemical evaluation for pituitary hormone deficiency may include a serum 8AM cortisol ± cosyntropin stimulation test, IGF-1, TSH and FT4, and LH/FSH/testosterone in men (or LH/FSH/estradiol in women who are not menstruating regularly).

## Management

The primary indication for more urgent surgical resection of a nonfunctioning pituitary adenoma is neurologic symptoms, including vision impairment. Transsphenoidal surgery may also be considered in cases of high risk of visual impairment (including a tumor close to the optic chiasm with plans for pregnancy), clinically significant tumor growth, and/or hypopituitarism. *Preoperatively*, hormone replacement for hypothyroidism, and especially for adrenal insufficiency, must be undertaken if present. *Perioperatively*, patients should be treated with stress dose glucocorticoids at the induction of anesthesia to cover the possibility of adrenal insufficiency should normal corticotroph cells be damaged during surgery. *Postoperatively*, monitoring for adrenal insufficiency, diabetes insipidus, and syndrome of inappropriate antidiuretic hormone (SIADH) is required. Patients should be treated with physiologic glucocorticoid replacement until adrenal insufficiency can be ruled out with an AM serum cortisol or a cosyntropin stimulation tests 6 weeks postoperatively. Postoperatively, patients should have their thirst, fluid intake and output, and serum sodium monitored in order to appropriately diagnose and treat diabetes insipidus and SIAD. This is typically done with serial serum sodiums on several days within the first two weeks after surgery. Patients may be seen back in clinic for repeat pituitary hormone evaluation 6 weeks postoperatively and repeat pituitary MRI scan 3–6 months postoperatively. Postoperative visual field and visual acuity testing should be scheduled for patients who had evidence of visual impairment preoperatively.

Transsphenoidal surgery is typically successful in reducing tumor volume and improving vision and is less successful in reversing hypopituitarism. One prospective observational cohort study and multiple retrospective studies have demonstrated residual tumor volume in 10–36% of patients, improved visual function in 75–91% of patients, and improved hypopituitarism in 35–50% of patients [12–14]. Even if there is little or no residual adenoma on pituitary MRI, the patient should still be monitored with serial pituitary MRI scans because approximately 20% of adenomas recur after transsphenoidal surgery [15], although the risk of recurrence is lower if there is no radiologic evidence of residual adenoma after surgery. If there is significant residual adenoma on pituitary MRI or progressive adenoma regrowth in the months or years after surgery, postoperative radiation therapy may be considered. When administered for adenoma regrowth, conventional radiation therapy results in 10-year control rates, defined as lack of clinical or radiologic progression, of approximately 80% [16]. However, patients who receive radiation therapy are at risk of developing hypopituitarism [17] and thus require long-term biochemical pituitary hormone monitoring. Currently, there are no approved pharmacologic treatment options for nonfunctioning pituitary adenomas. However, one historical cohort analysis suggested that dopamine agonist therapy in nonfunctioning pituitary adnenomas may be associated with decreased risk of tumor enlargement after transsphenoidal surgery [18]. This is biologically plausible given that most nonfunctioning pituitary adenomas express dopamine receptors.

There is insufficient evidence to make a recommendation regarding the primary treatment strategy for asymptomatic nonfunctioning pituitary adenomas. For those patients with nonfunctioning pituitary adenomas who do not undergo surgical resection, interval pituitary MRI imaging and biochemical evaluations should be performed. For some macroadenomas, pituitary MRI scan and biochemical evaluation for hypopituitarism may be repeated in 6 months and then 12 months thereafter if stability is demonstrated. For some microadenomas, pituitary MRI scan may be repeated in

12 months and then 12–24 months later if stability is demonstrated. Repeat biochemical evaluation for hypopituitarism may not be required for microadenomas if the patient's symptoms and MRI do not change over time. However, limited data are available on the natural history of nonfunctioning pituitary macroadenomas because most patients undergo surgery; studies suggest that approximately 40–50% of patients experience adenoma growth and 21–28.5% of patients eventually require surgery [19, 20].

## Outcome

This patient has a nonfunctioning pituitary macroadenoma that was diagnosed in the setting of pituitary hormone deficiency (central adrenal insufficiency). As he did not meet criteria for more urgent transsphenoidal surgery (i.e., neurological symptoms), he was monitored with serial pituitary MRI scans, visual field and visual acuity testing, and pituitary hormone biochemical evaluation. Over the course of 12 months, his sellar mass enlarged and came close to impinging on the optic chiasm. Given the time course of enlargement, the decision was made between the neurosurgeon, endocrinologist, and patient to undergo transsphenoidal surgery. The patient received stress dose glucocorticoids perioperatively. Pathology was consistent with a nonfunctioning pituitary adenoma. Postoperatively, the patient was discharged on physiologic glucocorticoid replacement and was monitored for the development of diabetes insipidus and/or SIADH, neither of which occurred. He will be seen in the neuroendocrine clinic for his 6-week postoperative visit.

**Clinical Pearls and Pitfalls**
- The most common presentations of nonfunctioning pituitary adenomas include neurologic symptoms (such as visual impairment), pituitary hormone deficiency due to mass effect from the adenoma, and an incidental sellar mass on an imaging study.

- In accordance with the Endocrine Society Clinical Practice Guidelines on Pituitary Incidentalomas, the evaluation of a newly diagnosed sellar mass >1 cm in size should include a detailed history and physical exam, a dedicated pituitary MRI, biochemical evaluation of pituitary hormone excess and deficiency, and visual field and visual acuity testing if clinically indicated.
- Although pituitary adenomas are the most common cause of a sellar mass >1 cm, the differential diagnosis is large and includes craniopharyngioma, meningioma, metastatic tumors, Rathke's cleft cyst, and hypophysitis, which is why a thorough evaluation is prudent.
- Hyperprolactinemia may be consequent to pituitary stalk compression by a sellar mass or due to a prolactinoma. In the former case, serum prolactin levels are typically <100 ng/mL, which can be used as a cutoff to help distinguish between stalk compression and a macroprolactinoma, the latter of which typically has serum prolactin levels >100 ng/mL. In patients with macroadenomas, the laboratory should measure serum prolactin levels in dilution to ensure that levels are not falsely lowered by a hook effect in the assay.
- Vision impairment due to optic chiasm compression is a clear indication for transsphenoidal surgery. Transsphenoidal surgery may also be considered in cases of high risk of visual impairment, clinically significant tumor growth, and/or hypopituitarism.
- Transsphenoidal surgery is typically successful in reducing tumor volume and improving vision and is less successful in reversing hypopituitarism. Even if there is little or no residual adenoma on pituitary MRI, the patient should still be monitored for recurrence with serial pituitary MRI scans. If there is significant residual adenoma on pituitary MRI or progressive adenoma regrowth after surgery, postoperative radiation therapy may be considered.

# References

1. Jukich PJ, McCarthy BJ, Surawicz TS, Freels S, Davis FG. Trends in incidence of primary brain tumors in the United States, 1985-1994. Neurooncology. 2001;3(3):141–51.
2. Popovic V, Damjanovic S. The effect of thyrotropin-releasing hormone on gonadotropin and free alpha-subunit secretion in patients with acromegaly and functionless pituitary tumors. Thyroid. 1998;8(10):935–9. https://doi.org/10.1089/thy.1998.8.935.
3. Rajasekaran S, Vanderpump M, Baldeweg S, et al. UK guidelines for the management of pituitary apoplexy. Clin Endocrinol (Oxf). 2011;74(1):9–20. https://doi.org/10.1111/j.1365-2265.2010.03913.x.
4. Fatemi N, Dusick JR, Mattozo C, et al. Pituitary hormonal loss and recovery after transsphenoidal adenoma removal. Neurosurgery. 2008;63(4):709–718; discussion 718–9. https://doi.org/10.1227/01.NEU.0000325725.77132.90.
5. Webb SM, Rigla M, Wägner A, Oliver B, Bartumeus F. Recovery of hypopituitarism after neurosurgical treatment of pituitary adenomas. J Clin Endocrinol Metab. 1999;84(10):3696–700. https://doi.org/10.1210/jcem.84.10.6019.
6. Marazuela M, Astigarraga B, Vicente A, et al. Recovery of visual and endocrine function following transsphenoidal surgery of large nonfunctioning pituitary adenomas. J Endocrinol Invest. 1994;17(9):703–7. https://doi.org/10.1007/BF03347763.
7. Dekkers OM, Pereira AM, Roelfsema F, et al. Observation alone after transsphenoidal surgery for nonfunctioning pituitary macroadenoma. J Clin Endocrinol Metab. 2006;91(5):1796–801. https://doi.org/10.1210/jc.2005-2552.
8. Molitch ME. Nonfunctioning pituitary tumors and pituitary incidentalomas. Endocrinol Metab Clin North Am. 2008;37(1):151–171, xi. https://doi.org/10.1016/j.ecl.2007.10.011.
9. Freda PU, Beckers AM, Katznelson L, et al. Pituitary incidentaloma: an Endocrine Society clinical practice guideline. J Clin Endocrinol Metab. 2011;96(4):894–904. https://doi.org/10.1210/jc.2010-1048.
10. Freda PU, Post KD. Differential diagnosis of sellar masses. Endocrinol Metab Clin North Am. 1999;28(1):81–117, vi.
11. Karavitaki N, Thanabalasingham G, Shore HCA, et al. Do the limits of serum prolactin in disconnection hyperprolactinaemia need re-definition? A study of 226 patients with histologically verified non-functioning pituitary macroadenoma. Clin Endocrinol (Oxf). 2006;65(4):524–9. https://doi.org/10.1111/j.1365-2265.2006.02627.x.
12. Chen L, White WL, Spetzler RF, Xu B. A prospective study of nonfunctioning pituitary adenomas: presentation, management, and clinical outcome. J Neurooncol. 2011;102(1):129–38. https://doi.org/10.1007/s11060-010-0302-x.

13. Dallapiazza RF, Grober Y, Starke RM, Laws ER, Jane JA. Long-term results of endonasal endoscopic transsphenoidal resection of nonfunctioning pituitary macroadenomas. Neurosurgery. 2015;76(1):42–52; discussion 52–3. https://doi.org/10.1227/NEU.0000000000000563.

14. Mortini P, Losa M, Barzaghi R, Boari N, Giovanelli M. Results of transsphenoidal surgery in a large series of patients with pituitary adenoma. Neurosurgery. 2005;56(6):1222–1233; discussion 1233.

15. Murad MH, Fernández-Balsells MM, Barwise A, et al. Outcomes of surgical treatment for nonfunctioning pituitary adenomas: a systematic review and meta-analysis. Clin Endocrinol (Oxf). 2010;73(6):777–91. https://doi.org/10.1111/j.1365-2265.2010.03875.x.

16. Woollons AC, Hunn MK, Rajapakse YR, et al. Non-functioning pituitary adenomas: indications for postoperative radiotherapy. Clin Endocrinol. 2000;53(6):713–7. https://doi.org/10.1046/j.1365-2265.2000.01153.x.

17. Boelaert K, Gittoes NJ. Radiotherapy for non-functioning pituitary adenomas. Eur J Endocrinol. 2001;144(6):569–75.

18. Greenman Y, Cooper O, Yaish I, et al. Treatment of clinically nonfunctioning pituitary adenomas with dopamine agonists. Eur J Endocrinol. 2016;175(1):63–72. https://doi.org/10.1530/EJE-16-0206.

19. Dekkers OM, Hammer S, de Keizer RJW, et al. The natural course of nonfunctioning pituitary macroadenomas. Eur J Endocrinol. 2007;156(2):217–24. https://doi.org/10.1530/eje.1.02334.

20. Arita K, Tominaga A, Sugiyama K, et al. Natural course of incidentally found nonfunctioning pituitary adenoma, with special reference to pituitary apoplexy during follow-up examination. J Neurosurg. 2006;104(6):884–91. https://doi.org/10.3171/jns.2006.104.6.884.

# Chapter 4
# Cushing's Disease: Common Pitfalls in Diagnosis

Pouneh K. Fazeli

## Case Presentation

A 59-year-old woman with a past medical history of hypertension and type 2 diabetes mellitus presented to her endocrinologist complaining of a one-year history of a 23 kg weight gain (current weight, 103.6 kg) and worsening control of her type 2 diabetes mellitus.

On review of systems, the patient noted easy bruising, thinning hair, and proximal muscle weakness, manifest as discomfort and difficulty walking up stairs. Her physical exam was notable for plethora, central obesity, a posterior cervical pad, supraclavicular fullness, and thinning skin. The endocrinologist ordered a basic metabolic panel, hemoglobin A1C, and two 24 hour (24-h) urine collections for free cortisol and creatinine. The laboratory panel was notable for a blood urea nitrogen (BUN) of 25 mg/dL (normal range, 8–25), a plasma creatinine of 1.44 (normal range, 0.60–1.50), and an estimated glomerular filtration rate (eGFR) of 37 mL/min/1.73 m$^2$ (normal range, $\geq 60$), as well as an elevated hemoglo-

P. K. Fazeli (✉)
Neuroendocrine Unit, Massachusetts General Hospital,
Harvard Medical School, Boston, MA, USA
e-mail: pkfazeli@partners.org

© Springer International Publishing AG, part of Springer Nature 2018     31
L. B. Nachtigall (ed.), *Pituitary Tumors*,
https://doi.org/10.1007/978-3-319-90909-7_4

bin A1C (8%). The two 24-h urine collections for free cortisol were notably normal [one with a free cortisol level of 29 μg/24 h (normal range, 4–50), a 24-h urine creatinine level of 1.08 g (normal range, 0.6–2.5 g/24 h), and a total collection volume of 2000 mL and the second with a 24-h urine free cortisol of 17.5 μg (normal range, 4–50), 24-h urine creatinine of 1 g (normal range, 0.6–2.5 g/24 h), and urine volume of 1650 mL]. The patient was referred for further evaluation.

## My Management

1. Given the clinical signs and symptoms of Cushing's, perform additional tests for Cushing's.

   (a) 1 mg dexamethasone suppression test
   (b) Late-night salivary cortisol measurement

2. If additional tests demonstrate hypercortisolemia, check an ACTH level to localize the source of cortisol production

## Assessment and Diagnosis

In 2008, the Endocrine Society published guidelines for establishing the diagnosis of Cushing's syndrome [1]. Three tests were recommended for initial testing of individuals suspected of having Cushing's syndrome: (1) 24-h urine free cortisol (two measurements), (2) late-night salivary cortisol (two measurements), and (3) low-dose dexamethasone suppression testing (either the 1 mg overnight dexamethasone suppression test or the longer 2 mg/day, 48 h dexamethasone suppression test). If the initial testing is suggestive of Cushing's, the guidelines recommend that a second test be performed for further confirmation [1]. While each of these tests has good diagnostic accuracy [2], there are a number of factors that may contribute to falsely normal or falsely abnormal results. Importantly, the decision to screen a patient for Cushing's should be carefully considered because certain populations are more at risk for having false-positive results. For example, approximately 25% of overweight or obese individuals without Cushing's may have an abnormal test result using one of the three first-line tests recommended by the Endocrine Society [3].

## Pitfalls in the Use of 24-h Urine Collection for Free Cortisol

A 24-h urine collection for free cortisol is a highly accurate screening tool for individuals suspected of having Cushing's syndrome [2]. Although a 24-h collection can sometimes be cumbersome for patients, it can be performed as an outpatient and dropped off at a laboratory making it potentially quite convenient. Importantly, the possible causes of false-positive and false-negative results should be considered prior to ordering a 24-h urine collection for free cortisol as an initial screening test.

**False-Negative Results**: As in the case above, excretion of cortisol may be abnormal in individuals with impaired renal function [4]. Importantly, even moderate reductions in renal function can lead to falsely low cortisol levels in a 24-h urine collection [5], and therefore this should be considered prior to ordering a 24-h urine collection for free cortisol and/or when interpreting the results of such testing. In the patient described above, the low eGFR and the fact that her 24 h urine creatinine levels were <15 mg/kg/24 h suggest that the results of the 24-h urine free cortisol testing may not be accurate.

**False-Positive Results**: Falsely elevated 24-h urine free cortisol levels may be seen in individuals who drink large amounts of fluid. A study investigating the effects of high fluid intake on cortisol excretion found that 23 out of 30 subjects had urine free cortisol levels above the normal range when drinking large amounts of fluid (mean urine volume: 3800 ± 1033 mL per day), but only 6 out of 30 of these individuals had abnormal results when drinking a normal amount of fluid (mean urine volume, 1070 ± 376 mL/day) [6]. Therefore, volume of fluid intake should be taken into consideration when evaluating an elevated 24-h urine free cortisol value.

## Pitfalls in the Use of Late-Night Salivary Cortisol Levels

Late-night salivary cortisol testing is a convenient and simple way of screening for hypercortisolemia. Patients can perform the testing at home by providing a saliva sample prior to bedtime (preferably between 11 pm and midnight). The kits can then be delivered or mailed back to a laboratory for analysis. While very convenient and very sensitive at detecting Cushing's [7, 8], false-positive test results are not uncommon in a number of populations.

A study of male veterans with a mean age of approximately 60 years demonstrated that false-positive results are common with increasing age and in those with type 2 diabetes mellitus [9]. In this group, which did not consist of any patients with known Cushing's syndrome, over 40% of patients who were 60 years of age or older with type 2 diabetes and hypertension had an abnormal late-night salivary cortisol level, suggesting that late-night salivary cortisol testing may not be a good initial test in this patient population [9]. This is likely due to the fact that the threshold for a normal value is based on young, healthy individuals [7] and therefore may be difficult to apply to an older population with comorbid conditions.

Another group in whom late-night salivary cortisol levels may be inaccurate is the night-shift worker. Cortisol secretion patterns change when sleep schedules are altered [10] and salivary cortisol profiles are different in nurses who work the night shift as compared to day shift workers [11]. Therefore the results of late-night salivary cortisol tests may be difficult to interpret in individuals who are night shift workers or in individuals who have rotating work schedules.

## Pitfalls in the Use of the Low-Dose Dexamethasone Suppression Test

The low-dose dexamethasone suppression test can be used to test the suppressibility of the hypothalamic-pituitary-adrenal axis and is an accurate means of evaluating for hypercortisolemia [2]. The 1 mg dexamethasone suppression test can be performed easily as an outpatient with the patient taking 1 mg of dexamethasone between 11 pm and 12 am at night and having a serum cortisol level drawn at 8 am the next morning. A cortisol level of <1.8 μg/dL is the recommended cutoff which makes the test highly sensitive and therefore reduces the likelihood of a false-negative result [1].

Since there are a number of medications which can accelerate the metabolism of dexamethasone and therefore lead to a false-positive result, checking a serum dexamethasone level in addition to a serum cortisol level at 8 am is instrumental in interpreting the results of testing. Medications that induce cytochrome P450 3A4, an oxidizing enzyme important for drug metabolism, accelerate the breakdown of dexamethasone, which may lead to a false-positive result. These drugs include antiseizure medications such as phenytoin and carbamazepine [12] as well as the antibiotic rifampin [13]. Women who are using oral contraceptives also may have a false-positive result with low-dose dexamethasone suppression testing because of the estrogen-associated increase in cortisol binding globulin [14, 15; therefore the oral contraceptive pill should be stopped at least 6 weeks before this test is performed.

## Management

Given the clinical signs and symptoms of Cushing's, I opted to perform a second test, a 1 mg overnight dexamethasone suppression test. The patient's 8 am post-dexamethasone cortisol level was 10.7 μg/dL (normal <1.8 μg/dL), and a dexamethasone level checked at the time of the 8 am blood draw was appropriate. Two late-night salivary cortisol levels were subsequently checked and both were elevated. An ACTH level was in the normal range (51 pg/mL with normal range, 6–76), and therefore ACTH-dependent Cushing's was diagnosed.

## Outcome

A pituitary MRI demonstrated a 6 mm sellar lesion, and inferior petrosal sinus sampling (IPSS) was performed, given the high prevalence rate of pituitary adenomas in the general population (estimated to be approximately 17%) [16] and the fact that the pituitary lesion was <1 cm in size. Importantly, the IPSS was performed on a day in which hypercortisolemia was confirmed (a late-night salivary cortisol level from the night before the IPSS was elevated), thus minimizing the potential for a false-positive result [17]. The IPSS results were consistent with a central source of ACTH production, and transsphenoidal surgery was subsequently performed. The pathology was notable for a pituitary adenoma with many tumor cells reactive for ACTH upon immunohistochemical staining.

**Clinical Pearls and Pitfalls**
- Establishing the diagnosis of Cushing's can be extremely challenging.
- The available screening tests for Cushing's are highly accurate, but careful consideration must be taken in choosing which test to perform in a given patient, given the possibility of a falsely abnormal or a falsely normal result.
- Individuals with reduced renal function may have falsely normal 24-h urine free cortisol levels.
- High fluid intake may result in a falsely elevated 24-h urine free cortisol level.
- A serum dexamethasone level should be checked at the same time as a cortisol level in patients undergoing dexamethasone suppression testing.

# References

1. Nieman LK, Biller BM, Findling JW, Newell-Price J, Savage MO, Stewart PM, Montori VM. The diagnosis of Cushing's syndrome: an Endocrine Society Clinical Practice Guideline. J Clin Endocrinol Metab. 2008;93:1526–40.
2. Elamin MB, Murad MH, Mullan R, Erickson D, Harris K, Nadeem S, Ennis R, Erwin PJ, Montori VM. Accuracy of diagnostic tests for Cushing's syndrome: a systematic review and metaanalyses. J Clin Endocrinol Metab. 2008;93:1553–62.
3. Baid SK, Rubino D, Sinaii N, Ramsey S, Frank A, Nieman LK. Specificity of screening tests for Cushing's syndrome in an overweight and obese population. J Clin Endocrinol Metab. 2009;94:3857–64.
4. Sederberg-Olsen P, Binder C, Kehlet H. Urinary excretion of free cortisol in impaired renal function. Acta Endocrinol (Copenh). 1975;78:86–90.
5. Chan KC, Lit LC, Law EL, Tai MH, Yung CU, Chan MH, Lam CW. Diminished urinary free cortisol excretion in patients with moderate and severe renal impairment. Clin Chem. 2004;50:757–9.
6. Mericq MV, Cutler GB Jr. High fluid intake increases urine free cortisol excretion in normal subjects. J Clin Endocrinol Metab. 1998;83:682–4.
7. Raff H, Raff JL, Findling JW. Late-night salivary cortisol as a screening test for Cushing's syndrome. J Clin Endocrinol Metab. 1998;83:2681–6.
8. Putignano P, Toja P, Dubini A, Pecori Giraldi F, Corsello SM, Cavagnini F. Midnight salivary cortisol versus urinary free and midnight serum cortisol as screening tests for Cushing's syndrome. J Clin Endocrinol Metab. 2003;88:4153–7.
9. Liu H, Bravata DM, Cabaccan J, Raff H, Ryzen E. Elevated late-night salivary cortisol levels in elderly male type 2 diabetic veterans. Clin Endocrinol (Oxf). 2005;63:642–9.
10. Rehman JU, Brismar K, Holmback U, Akerstedt T, Axelsson J. Sleeping during the day: effects on the 24-h patterns of IGF-binding protein 1, insulin, glucose, cortisol, and growth hormone. Eur J Endocrinol. 2010;163:383–90.
11. Niu SF, Chung MH, Chu H, Tsai JC, Lin CC, Liao YM, Ou KL, O'Brien AP, Chou KR. Differences in cortisol profiles and circadian adjustment time between nurses working night shifts and regular day shifts: a prospective longitudinal study. Int J Nurs Stud. 2015;52:1193–201.
12. Perucca E. Clinically relevant drug interactions with antiepileptic drugs. Br J Clin Pharmacol. 2006;61:246–55.
13. Kyriazopoulou V, Vagenakis AG. Abnormal overnight dexamethasone suppression test in subjects receiving rifampicin therapy. J Clin Endocrinol Metab. 1992;75:315–7.
14. Blethen SL, Chasalow FI. Overnight dexamethasone suppression test: normal responses and the diagnosis of Cushing's syndrome. Steroids. 1989;54:185–93.

15. Nickelsen T, Lissner W, Schoffling K. The dexamethasone suppression test and long-term contraceptive treatment: measurement of ACTH or salivary cortisol does not improve the reliability of the test. Exp Clin Endocrinol. 1989;94:275–80.
16. Ezzat S, Asa SL, Couldwell WT, Barr CE, Dodge WE, Vance ML, McCutcheon IE. The prevalence of pituitary adenomas: a systematic review. Cancer. 2004;101:613–9.
17. Yamamoto Y, Davis DH, Nippoldt TB, Young WF Jr, Huston J 3rd, Parisi JE. False-positive inferior petrosal sinus sampling in the diagnosis of Cushing's disease. Report of two cases. J Neurosurg. 1995;83:1087–91.

# Chapter 5
# Management of Cushing's Disease

**Dariush Jahandideh and Nicholas A. Tritos**

## Case Presentation

A 24-year-old woman presented to her primary care physician for evaluation of oligomenorrhea and obesity. Her menses had started at age 12 years and had been regular on a monthly basis until 2 years before her presentation. Subsequently, she noted that menses occurred every 2–3 months with diminished flow. She gained 40 lb over 2 years despite receiving nutrition counseling and making efforts to limit her caloric intake. On review of systems, she reported persistent fatigue, facial rounding, spontaneous bruising without trauma, and facial acne. She had been previously healthy and was taking no medications. She had used no glucocorticoids, never smoked, and was drinking no alcohol. She was working as an accountant and had recently married. She was anxious to start a family soon.

On examination, her blood pressure was abnormally high on several occasions (150/95–160/98 mmHg). Her weight was 210 lb with a height of 65 inches (BMI, 34.9 kg/m$^2$). There was facial rounding, mild plethora, and acne present on examination. There were 5–6-mm-wide purple striae present on the abdomen and flanks. Proximal muscle strength was normal.

D. Jahandideh · N. A. Tritos (✉)
Neuroendocrine Unit, Massachusetts General Hospital,
Harvard Medical School, Boston, MA, USA
e-mail: djahandideh@mgh.harvard.edu; ntritos@mgh.harvard.edu

© Springer International Publishing AG, part of Springer Nature 2018     39
L. B. Nachtigall (ed.), *Pituitary Tumors*,
https://doi.org/10.1007/978-3-319-90909-7_5

Laboratory tests showed normal serum electrolytes, creatinine, and fasting glucose. Her 24-h urine free cortisol (UFC) was 269 μg/24 h (normal, 3.5–45) and 207 μg/24 h in two different collections (both with normal urine creatinine and volume). Two late-night salivary cortisol test results were 21.8 nmol/L (normal, 0.3–4.3) and 8.7 nmol/L, respectively. Plasma corticotropin (ACTH) level was 68 pg/mL (normal, 4–70). Pituitary magnetic resonance imaging (MRI) showed a 4 mm sellar hypodensity. She underwent bilateral inferior petrosal sinus sampling (BIPSS), which showed a central ACTH gradient (peak central to peripheral ACTH ratio = 5:1), diagnostic of Cushing's disease (CD).

She underwent transsphenoidal surgery (TSS) by an experienced pituitary neurosurgeon. Pathology showed a pituitary adenoma, which was positive for ACTH on immunostaining. Postoperatively, her early morning serum cortisol was not low (15–19 μg/dL), measured on several occasions within the first postoperative week, and her 24 h UFC also remained elevated (108–142 μg/24 h) on several occasions, indicating that she was not in remission.

Approximately 8 weeks after the first TSS, she underwent a second pituitary operation in the hope of achieving remission. No tumor was found and she remained hypercortisolemic postoperatively. Treatment with metyrapone was begun at a dose of 250 mg by mouth three times daily. However, the patient developed nausea and dizziness and had to discontinue the medication within 1 week. Treatment with cabergoline was then started at a dose of 0.5 mg by mouth weekly. However, the medication was also discontinued after 2 weeks because of persistent nausea and dizziness. She declined radiation therapy to the sella.

## Our Management Options

1. Pasireotide
2. Mitotane
3. Bilateral adrenalectomy
4. Mifepristone

# Management of Cushing's Disease

The first-line treatment of CD is TSS by an experienced pituitary surgeon, which controls hypercortisolism rapidly and effectively with a low risk of hypopituitarism following surgery [1].

The outcome of TSS depends on different factors, including surgeon's level of experience, tumor size and extension into adjacent structures, and recognition of the tumor before surgery on pituitary MRI, intraoperatively, or on pathologic examination [2, 3].

Results of several studies suggest that the success rate of the first TSS in CD is 70–90% in patients with intrasellar microadenomas who are operated on by experienced pituitary neurosurgeons [4]. If TSS does not lead to remission of hypercortisolism or if recurrence occurs (the latter developing in up to 30% of patients on long-term follow-up), then second-line treatment can be a second TSS, especially if the first one was not done by an experienced pituitary surgeon. After repeat TSS, about 50–70% of CD patients with recurrent or persistent disease will be in remission [5, 6].

In those patients who have failed TSS or are not surgical candidates, a reasonable next option is radiation therapy to the sella. Based on reports from different studies, the success rate of radiation therapy in controlling hypercortisolism is up to 86% of patients. In addition, tumor growth is controlled in 90–100% of patients [7, 8]. Unlike TSS, it can take a long time (from 6 months to 10 years) for endocrine remission to occur after radiation therapy. In addition, this treatment carries a high risk of anterior hypopituitarism. After radiation therapy, the 5-year cumulative risk of hypopituitarism is 30–40%, which likely increases over time [8, 9].

Patients who have received radiation therapy require medical therapy to control hypercortisolism until radiation therapy takes effect. There are several medical options that act on different areas of the hypothalamic-pituitary-adrenal axis, including adrenal steroidogenesis inhibitors, centrally acting agents, and glucocorticoid receptor antagonists. All medications require careful dose titration and long-term monitoring to detect and mitigate hypoadrenalism, which may develop as an extension of their desired effects.

Steroidogenesis inhibitors are effective in controlling cortisol production by the adrenal glands. As they lower serum cortisol, the negative feedback on the hypothalamus and pituitary gland is attenuated. Thus, after a while there might be an escape from the effect of the medication.

Ketoconazole is a steroidogenesis inhibitor that acts by blocking several steroidogenic enzymes and is effective in controlling cortisol levels in 50–70% of patients. Its adverse effects include gastrointestinal (GI) symptoms, rash, gynecomastia, or potentially serious hepatotoxicity. Ketoconazole is preferred over metyrapone in women [10]. Ketoconazole is FDA category C and is not recommended during pregnancy because it often decreases testosterone levels and could potentially interfere with masculinization of a male fetus. However, it has been used in a few pregnant women without reports of fetal harm, despite its potential antiandrogenic effects [11–13].

Metyrapone inhibits 11-beta hydroxylase and controls cortisol levels in up to 75% of patients. This agent leads to accumulation of androgenic precursors, which may often cause hirsutism in women. There are also other possible adverse effects, including GI symptoms, rash, dizziness, hypertension, and edema. Metyrapone is the most frequently used medication during pregnancy [14]. Metyrapone seems generally well tolerated during pregnancy, although caution is advised with the use of any medication in pregnancy [15]. It has not been associated with fetal developmental or maternal hepatotoxic adverse effects [3].

Mitotane has a significantly slower onset of action compared to other agents. It inhibits multiple steroidogenic enzymes and is adrenolytic in high doses. Mitotane has many possible adverse effects, including GI and neurologic symptoms. This agent is stored in adipose tissue where it can remain for several years after discontinuation. Since it can cross the placenta and is teratogenic, it should not be used in women who are planning to conceive in the next 5 years [16, 17].

The only steroidogenesis inhibitor that is available for intravenous use is etomidate, which causes rapid reduction in serum cortisol levels. This agent may cause excessive sedation [18]. Aminoglutethimide and trilostane are two other steroidogenesis inhibitors that are no longer available in the USA [4].

Centrally acting agents are another class of medications that can be used in CD. Cabergoline, a dopamine agonist that is approved by the FDA for the treatment of hyperprolactinemia, has been reported to be effective in controlling hypercortisolism in 30–40% of patients with CD. The effect of cabergoline in these patients is predicated by the frequent expression of dopamine 2 receptors in pituitary tumor cells of patients with CD [19]. The dose range of cabergoline reported in studies of patients with CD is relatively high (0.5–7 mg per week) in comparison with the usual doses, ranging between 0.5 and 2.0 mg per week, used in hyperprolactinemia. Adverse effects may include nausea, orthostasis, and, less often, headache, constipation, anxiety, depression, impulsivity, or exacerbation of psychosis [4]. In addition, cabergoline use in high doses has been associated with cardiac valvulopathy in patients with Parkinson's disease. Cabergoline use has been reported in small numbers of hyperprolactinemic women during pregnancy, but has not been studied in pregnant women with CD.

Pasireotide is a somatostatin receptor ligand with affinity for multiple somatostatin receptor isoforms (SSR 1, 2, 3, and 5). SSR5 is often expressed by pituitary tumor cells in patients with CD. This agent is approved by the FDA for use in patients with CD, wherein it may control hypercortisolism in 20–30% of patients [20]. Adverse effects may include GI toxicity, gallstones, and hyperglycemia (including diabetes mellitus). There have been no studies of pasireotide in pregnant women.

Another means of controlling the effects of hypercortisolism is to block the glucocorticoid receptor. Mifepristone is a progesterone receptor and type 2 glucocorticoid receptor antagonist, which can lead to improvements in overall clinical status, decrease in weight, and hyperglycemia in most treated patients. However, mifepristone has to be titrated based on clinical criteria alone and can cause several adverse effects, including hypokalemia, hypertension, and endometrial hyperplasia. In addition, mifepristone will terminate pregnancy [21]. With the exception of mifepristone and pasireotide, medications used to treat CD are used "off label" in the USA (i.e., without an FDA-approved indication for CD).

## The Role of Bilateral Adrenalectomy in Cushing's Disease

Before refinement of pituitary surgery, bilateral adrenalectomy was widely used as a first-line treatment for CD. As other effective treatment options evolved, bilateral adrenalectomy is currently reserved for those who have either failed or are not candidates for TSS, radiation therapy, or medical therapy [4]. Patients with severe CD who have failed TSS and cannot be controlled on medical therapy may particularly benefit from bilateral adrenalectomy, which generally affords prompt control of hypercortisolism. In addition, female patients planning to conceive who have failed TSS may be considered for bilateral adrenalectomy, particularly if they wish to avoid the risk of anterior hypopituitarism associated with radiation therapy.

Bilateral adrenalectomy rapidly eliminates hypercortisolism in almost all patients. However, this procedure will also cause permanent adrenal insufficiency necessitating lifelong glucocorticoid and mineralocorticoid replacement. Nelson's syndrome is another possible complication that might occur in CD patients after bilateral adrenalectomy as a consequence of loss of feedback inhibition exerted by cortisol on tumorous corticotrophs. Nelson's syndrome may develop in 8–38% of the patients after bilateral adrenalectomy in different reports and involves progressive growth of corticotroph tumors that can become locally invasive causing mass effect as well as diffuse skin hyperpigmentation as a result of tumorous oversecretion of melanotropic peptides [22].

In a study of quality of life of 39 patients who underwent laparoscopic bilateral adrenalectomy as a treatment for CD, the majority of patients had significant improvement in their symptoms and reported their quality of life as being comparable to that of patients treated by TSS [23].

# Morbidity and Mortality Associated with Hypercortisolism During Pregnancy

Hypercortisolism frequently leads to hypogonadism, which interferes with normal follicular development and ovulation. Accordingly, it is rare for women with active hypercortisolism to conceive. Case series of women with hypercortisolism diagnosed during pregnancy have found a substantial risk of maternal morbidity (70% of pregnant women with this condition) and mortality. These women are at increased risk of diabetes mellitus, hypertension, and less frequently osteoporosis, fractures, poor wound healing, severe psychiatric complications, maternal cardiac failure, and death. Hypercortisolism is also linked to serious fetal adverse effects, including spontaneous abortion, intrauterine growth retardation, prematurity, stillbirth, and intrauterine death [15]. Fetal adrenal insufficiency is rare, and there has been no report of signs of glucocorticoid excess in newborns delivered by women with hypercortisolism. The fetus is mostly protected from the adverse effects of hypercortisolism as a consequence of degradation of cortisol by placental tissue. The fetal adverse effects caused by cortisol excess are probably caused by induced maternal and placental abnormalities [15, 24].

During pregnancy, adrenal causes of hypercortisolism appear to be more prevalent, and CD is less common than in non-gravid patients, possibly because CD patients are more hyperandrogenic compared to those with adrenal adenomas [24].

Prompt treatment that leads to rapid control of hypercortisolism is advisable during pregnancy. A study of 136 pregnancies showed that pregnant women who received treatment at a mean gestational age of 20 ± 1 weeks gave birth to 50 infants (89%), while those with no treatment for their hypercortisolemia had 59 live births (76%). In this study, surgical treatment of hypercortisolism was suggested as first-line treatment and medical therapy as a second-line option during pregnancy [15]. Adrenalectomy is likely effective in these patients, wherein the live birth rate was 87% among those who underwent unilateral or bilateral adrenalectomy, depending on the underlying etiology of hypercortisolism [24].

## Treatment Options in Women with Cushing's Disease Planning to Conceive

Pituitary surgery is generally a first-line treatment in women with CD planning to conceive. However, if CD persists or recurs after up to two pituitary operations, then radiation therapy with interim medical therapy can be considered. Radiation therapy may lead to anterior hypopituitarism, necessitating the use of assisted reproductive technologies in this population.

Of note, CD patients who are planning to conceive are not candidates for some of the medical treatment options due to potential adverse effects on the fetus. Ketoconazole has been shown to cross the placenta in rats and has teratogenic and abortifacient effects. However, there are some reports of pregnant CD patients who received ketoconazole without evident harm. In general, ketoconazole is best avoided during preconception or pregnancy due to the potential risk of interference with masculinization of a male fetus. Mitotane is teratogenic. This agent is stored in adipose tissue for several years and should be stopped 5 years before the patient intends to conceive. Mifepristone will terminate pregnancy and should obviously be avoided in preconception. Pasireotide is labeled by the FDA as a category C drug, and there are no studies of its use in pregnant women [4].

Metyrapone is the most widely used medication in pregnant CD patients or those planning to conceive [24]. Cabergoline use has been reported in hyperprolactinemic women, but has not been specifically studied during preconception or pregnancy in CD.

# Outcome

Our patient had persistent CD after two pituitary operations, and she could not tolerate two medical therapies (metyrapone or cabergoline). She declined radiation therapy and opted for bilateral adrenalectomy. Postoperatively, she was placed on hydrocortisone (titrated to a maintenance dose of 10 mg in the morning and 5 mg in the early afternoon) and fludrocortisone (100 µg by mouth daily). Her menses resumed on a regular basis, hypertension resolved, and features of hypercortisolism gradually cleared. She lost 30 lb and was able to conceive naturally. Her hydrocortisone replacement dose was increased (to 15 mg in the morning and 5 mg in the early afternoon) during pregnancy, which was overall uneventful. She received stress dose glucocorticoid coverage during labor, and she delivered a healthy baby girl at term. A pituitary MRI examination was obtained at 8 weeks postpartum and showed no evident sellar mass.

**Clinical Pearls and Pitfalls**

- First-line treatment in patients with Cushing's disease is transsphenoidal surgery (TSS) by an experienced neurosurgeon. Surgery is effective in controlling hypercortisolism in 70–90% of patients (among those with an intrasellar microadenoma).

- Second-line treatment may involve repeat TSS, which has a success rate of 50–70%. High failure rates of a second TSS suggest the need for further treatments to manage this disease.

- Radiation therapy is a reasonable option in patients who have already failed surgery or are not candidates for surgery. The caveats of this modality are the relatively long time needed before its therapeutic effects are seen and the substantial risk of anterior hypopituitarism.

- There are several medications that can control Cushing's disease by different mechanisms, including steroidogenesis inhibitors, centrally acting agents, and glucocorticoid receptor antagonists. Medications are generally used as a "bridge" in patients who are awaiting the salutary effects of radiation therapy. The choice of the most suitable medication for each patient is empiric.

- Metyrapone is the most commonly used agent to control hypercortisolism during gestation. Several other medications, including mitotane and mifepristone, are contraindicated during preconception or gestation.

- The last resort for the management of patients with Cushing's disease is bilateral adrenalectomy. This procedure is usually done laparoscopically. Once the adrenal glands are removed, the patient should have tight adherence to replacement therapies, since severe adrenal insufficiency without steroid replacement is fatal.

# References

1. Nieman LK, Biller BM, Findling JW, Murad MH, Newell-Price J, Savage MO, Tabarin A. Treatment of Cushing's syndrome: an endocrine society clinical practice guideline. J Clin Endocrinol Metabol. 2015;100(8):2807–31.
2. Swearingen B, Biller BM, Barker FG, Katznelson L, Grinspoon S, Klibanski A, Zervas NT. Long-term mortality after transsphenoidal surgery for Cushing disease. Ann Intern Med. 1999;130(10):821–4.
3. Barker FG, Klibanski A, Swearingen B. Transsphenoidal surgery for pituitary tumors in the United States, 1996–2000: mortality, morbidity, and the effects of hospital and surgeon volume. J Clin Endocrinol Metabol. 2003;88(10):4709–19.
4. Tritos NA, Biller BM, Swearingen B. Management of Cushing disease. Nat Rev Endocrinol. 2011;7(5):279–89.
5. Esposito F, Dusick JR, Cohan P, Moftakhar P, McArthur D, Wang C, Swerdloff RS, Kelly DF. Early morning cortisol levels as a predictor of remission after transsphenoidal surgery for Cushing's disease. J Clin Endocrinol Metabol. 2006;91(1):7–13.
6. Ram Z, Nieman LK, Cutler GB Jr, Chrousos GP, Doppman JL, Oldfield EH. Early repeat surgery for persistent Cushing's disease. J Neurosurg. 1994;80(1):37–45.
7. Minniti G, Osti M, Jaffrain-Rea ML, Esposito V, Cantore G, Enrici RM. Long-term follow-up results of postoperative radiation therapy for Cushing's disease. J Neurooncol. 2007;84(1):79–84.
8. Petit JH, Biller BM, Yock TI, Swearingen B, Coen JJ, Chapman P, Ancukiewicz M, Bussiere M, Klibanski A, Loeffler JS. Proton stereotactic radiotherapy for persistent adrenocorticotropin-producing adenomas. J Clin Endocrinol Metabol. 2008;93(2):393–9.
9. Feigl GC, Bonelli CM, Berghold A, Mokry M. Effects of gamma knife radiosurgery of pituitary adenomas on pituitary function. J Neurosurg. 2002;97:415–21.
10. Sonino N, Boscaro M, Paoletta A, Mantero F, Zillotto D. Ketoconazole treatment in Cushing's syndrome: experience in 34 patients. Clin Endocrinol (Oxf). 1991;35(4):347–52.
11. Berwaerts J, Verhelst J, Mahler C, Abs R. Cushing's syndrome in pregnancy treated by ketoconazole: case report and review of the literature. Gynecol Endocrinol. 1999;13(3):175–82.
12. Amado JA, Pesquera C, Gonzalez EM, Otero M, Freijanes J, Alvarez A. Successful treatment with ketoconazole of Cushing's syndrome in pregnancy. Postgrad Med J. 1990;66(773):221–3.
13. Prebtani AP, Donat D, Ezzat S. Worrisome striae. Lancet. 2000;355(9216):1692.
14. Verhelst JA, Trainer PJ, Howlett TA, Perry L, Rees LH, Grossman AB, Wass JA, Sesser GM. Short and long-term responses to metyrapone in

the medical management of 91 patients with Cushing's syndrome. Clin Endocrinol (Oxf). 1991;35(2):169–78.

15. Lindsay JR, Jonklaas J, Oldfield EH, Nieman LK. Cushing's syndrome during pregnancy: personal experience and review of the literature. J Clin Endocrinol Metabol. 2005;90(5):3077–83.

16. Luton JP, Mahoudeau JA, Bouchard PH, Thieblot PH, Hautecouverture M, Simon D, Laudat MH, Touitou Y, Bricaire H. Treatment of Cushing's disease by o,p' DDD: survey of 62 cases. N Engl J Med. 1979;300(9):459–64.

17. Leiba S, Weinstein R, Shindel B, Lapidot M, Stern E, Levavi H, Rusecki Y, Abramovici A. The protracted effect of o,p'-DDD in Cushing's disease and its impact on adrenal morphogenesis of young human embryo. Ann Endocrinol. 1989;50(1):49–53.

18. Schulte HM, Benker G, Reinwein D, Sippell WG, Allolio B. Infusion of low dose etomidate: correction of hypercortisolemia in patients with Cushing's syndrome and dose-response relationship in normal subjects. J Clin Endocrinol Metabol. 1990;70(5):1426–30.

19. Godbout A, Manavela M, Danilowicz K, Beauregard H, Bruno OD, Lacroix A. Cabergoline monotherapy in the long-term treatment of Cushing's disease. Eur J Endocrinol. 2010;163(5):709–16.

20. Petersenn S, Salgado LR, Schopohl J, Portocarrero-Ortiz L, Arnaldi G, Lacroix A, Scaroni C, Ravichandran S, Kandra A, Biller BM. Long-term treatment of Cushing's disease with pasireotide: 5-year results from an open-label extension study of a Phase III trial. Endocrine. 2017;57(1):156–65.

21. Castinetti F, Fassnacht M, Johanssen S, Terzolo M, Bouchard P, Chanson P, Do Cao C, Morange I, Pico A, Ouzounian S, Young J. Merits and pitfalls of mifepristone in Cushing's syndrome. Eur J Endocrinol. 2009;160(6):1003–10.

22. Vik-Mo EO, Øksnes M, Pedersen PH, Wentzel-Larsen T, Rødahl E, Thorsen F, Schreiner T, Aanderud S, Lund-Johansen M. Gamma knife stereotactic radiosurgery of Nelson syndrome. Eur J Endocrinol. 2009;160(2):143–8.

23. Thompson SK, Hayman AV, Ludlam WH, Deveney CW, Loriaux DL, Sheppard BC. Improved quality of life after bilateral laparoscopic adrenalectomy for Cushing's disease: a 10-year experience. Ann Surg. 2007;245(5):790.

24. Lindsay JR, Nieman LK. The hypothalamic-pituitary-adrenal axis in pregnancy: challenges in disease detection and treatment. Endocr Rev. 2005;26(6):775–99.

# Chapter 6
# Acromegaly: Diagnosis and Management in Patients Who Present with Discrepancy Between IGF-1 and GH

Lisa B. Nachtigall

## Case Presentation

This is a woman who initially presented with galactorrhea at age 18 years and was found to have an elevated prolactin of 75 (normal <20 ng/mL). She reported progressive headaches, increase in nose size, increasing ring and shoe size, and swelling of fingers. On exam her vital signs were normal. She stood at 63 in. with a weight of 125 lb, blood pressure of 110/80, and heart rate of 72. Notable exam findings included an absence of the typical facial features of acromegaly except for a subtle increase in her nose and chin size compared to old photographs and a larger tongue. She had enlargement of feet and hands and thickened fingers. Visual field exam was normal, and the remainder of the exam was unremarkable. Biochemical testing revealed insulin growth factor 1 (IGF-1) was in the upper normal range at 624 (normal range 182–780 ng/mL) and a random growth hormone (GH) was 14 ng/mL. GH nadir on oral glucose tolerance test (OGTT) was

L. B. Nachtigall (✉)
Neuroendocrine Unit, Massachusetts General Hospital,
Harvard Medical School, Boston, MA, USA
e-mail: lnachtigall@partners.org

© Springer International Publishing AG, part of Springer Nature 2018     51
L. B. Nachtigall (ed.), *Pituitary Tumors*,
https://doi.org/10.1007/978-3-319-90909-7_6

Coronal                                        Sagittal

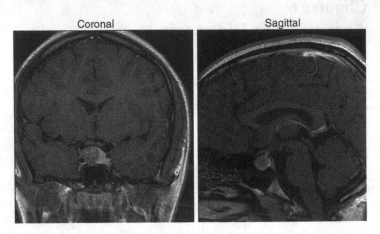

**Fig. 6.1** Pituitary MRI post contrast

high at 7.2 ng/mL, where normal OGTT nadir is <1 ng/mL. Morning cortisol and thyroid hormone levels were normal, and repeated prolactin (diluted) was again mildly elevated at 51.3 (0–20 ng/mL). Cosyntropin stimulation was normal, excluding adrenal insufficiency. Fasting glucose and hemoglobin AIc were normal. An MRI of the pituitary was ordered, which revealed a sellar mass approximately 1.4 cm in size without compression of the chiasm (Fig. 6.1).

Given her elevated GH and a macroadenoma, she underwent transsphenoidal surgery by an experienced pituitary surgery. A GH-secreting adenoma was confirmed on pathology which also showed rare prolactin-secreting cells. Six weeks postoperatively, she felt well and reported decrease in ring size. Pituitary MRI six weeks after surgery revealed a small lateral superior remnant of tumor, which the neurosurgeon determined to be likely accessible with repeat surgery. Twelve weeks postoperatively, after the second surgery, her menses became regular and IGF-1 improved at 463 (normal range 182–780 ng/mL). Nadir GH by OGTT, while improved, remained high at 4.3 ng/mL, where normal OGTT nadir is <1 ng/mL.

## My Management

1. A repeat surgery was recommended and performed by an expert pituitary surgeon.

   *We considered repeat pituitary surgery versus medical therapy with somatostatin analog, cabergoline, or pegvisomant. Given her young age, uncertainty of ongoing access to medical insurance coverage for drugs, and the fact that the tumor remnant was deemed likely to be accessible with a second surgery, after discussion of options and risks and benefits of each, a second surgery was recommended and the patient agreed.*

2. A postoperative MRI and anterior pituitary function tests were obtained.

3. Clinical assessment for signs and symptoms of acromegaly and biochemical testing for GH excess: OGTT for GH and IGF-1 levels were obtained at 6–12 weeks postoperatively.

4. A colonoscopy was suggested.

## Assessment and Diagnosis

The diagnosis of acromegaly is based on signs and symptoms of acromegaly and biochemical evidence of GH excess: a high GH and/or high IGF-1. The presence of pituitary tumor is visible on MRI in >90% of cases, and most of these, approximately 70% are macroadenomas [1]. This patient was originally thought to have a prolactinoma because her first presentation to her gynecologist was for galactorrhea. When she was seen by neuroendocrine, she was found to have subtle features of acromegaly, high GH but normal IGF-1, and ultimately pathology confirmed a GH-secreting macroadenoma.

Why was her IGF-1 normal if she had acromegaly, and what are the causes for the discrepancy between IGF-1 and GH? Possible reasons for a lower IGF-1 include exogenous estrogen, liver disease, starvation/malnourishment, and poorly controlled DM [2]. None of these applied in her case. She may have been restricting calories but was not known to have anorexia. Another possibility includes a range of problems with IGF-1 assays [3]. In this case, the normal range for her age was up to 780 ng/mL, and this may have been inappropriately high, placing her fairly high level of 624 within the normal range. GH may be elevated in anorexia, normal puberty, pregnancy, diabetes mellitus and hypoglycemia, liver disease, and exogenous estrogen [4]. These conditions should be considered if IGF-1 is normal in the setting of high GH or the clinical diagnosis is in question; but none of these explained the high GH in this case of isolated GH excess, and ultimately pathology confirmed acromegaly.

She was only 18 years at her first presentation of acromegaly. The mean age at diagnosis is typically in the fourth decade, and most patients have had already had the disease for 7–10 years prior to diagnosis [1]. Younger patients are more likely to have more aggressive disease and more likely to have germ-line aryl hydro-carbon receptor-interacting protein (AIP) mutations even in the absence of known family history [5]. Gigantism occurs when the GH excess begins before the pubertal closure of the epiphyses. At 63 inches, she was not tall relative to her mid-parental height because menarche and puberty had been completed before the onset of the acromegaly, and therefore she presumably had closure of her epiphyses prior to the onset of acromegaly.

At the time of diagnosis of acromegaly, assessment should include evaluations of comorbidities associated with acromegaly. These include evaluation of glucose and hemoglobin A1C to screen for diabetes or glucose intolerance, a test for sleep apnea if there are suggestive symptoms, an echocardiogram if there are cardiac symptoms, and a screening colonoscopy to evaluate for colonic polyps and colon cancer [6]. In addition, testing anterior hormonal function to assess for co-secretion or deficiencies is indicated at baseline and after surgical therapy [7]. Visual field testing is appro-priate in patients with MRI evidence of tumors which contact or invade the optic chiasm and preconception in reproductive age patients with macroadenomas [6].

# Management

Pituitary surgery remains a first-line therapy for acromegaly unless contraindicated, refused, inaccessible, or if there is no compression of chiasm and patients are unlikely to be surgically cured; in these cases primary medical therapy is appropriate [6].

Medical therapy includes cabergoline, somatostatin analogs (SSAs), and GH receptor antagonist [8]. Cabergoline is more likely to be effective as monotherapy if the IGF-1 is less than double normal and typically has minimal effect on tumor reduction [9]. Dopamine agonists such as cabergoline are generally well tolerated but can increase impulsive behavior rarely and must be avoided in patients with psychotic disorders as they may stimulate psychosis in such patients [10, 11]. The first-generation somatostatin analogs include lanreotide and octreotide, target somatostatin subtype receptors (SSTR) 2 and 5, and are available as long-acting monthly injections, which decrease GH excess and control tumor in 20–70% of patients. Side effects may include diarrhea, nausea, abdominal pain, gallstones, diabetes, injection site pain, and rarely hypoglycemia, bradycardia, and hair loss. Pasireotide, a second-generation somatostatin analog, binds to SSTR 1, 2, 3, and 5 and has slightly greater efficacy in controlling GH excess and also confers tumor control in responsive patients with a side effect profile similar to a first-generation SSA but with increased risk of diabetes and hyperglycemia. Pegvisomant, a growth hormone receptor antagonist, does not typically decrease tumor but effectively controls IGF-1 in most patients with minimal side effects: rarely causing increase in liver enzymes, headaches, hives, or lipohypertrophy at injection sites. If monotherapy is not effective, then therapies can be combined: SSA plus pegvisomant, SSA plus cabergoline, and cabergoline plus SSA.

If medical therapies are not tolerated or inaccessible, radiation is an option. Gamma knife or proton beam can be given as a single dose unless the tumor is very near the optic chiasm, in which case single-dose radiotherapy cannot be used, and traditional fractionated radiation therapy can be given over many weeks. Since radiotherapy takes 2–20 years to produce a remission [12], medical therapy must be used until then to control GH excess.

## Outcome

The first surgery was not effective but was uncomplicated and improved GH and IGF-1 levels and symptoms. The second surgery was not curative but associated with further improvement of GH. Patient could not tolerate the SSA due to nausea and weight loss. She could not tolerate cabergoline due to fatigue and mood changes. She had radiation therapy and was observed off medications since her IGF-1 was normal, and she did not have symptoms of acromegaly. However, for several years without medical insurance, she was lost to follow-up. Three years after radiotherapy, her IGF-1 began to rise, and signs and symptoms of acromegaly progressed including thickening of the fingers, joint pain, headaches,

| **Table 6.1** Symptoms and signs of acromegaly | |
|---|---|
| | Excessive sweating |
| | Headache |
| | Arthralgia |
| | Arthritis |
| | Enlargement hands or feet |
| | Change in ring size, hat size, or shoe size |
| | New spaces between teeth |
| | Jaw growth/prognathism |
| | Galactorrhea |
| | Coarsening of facial features |
| | Hoarseness or gravelly voice |
| | Large tongue |
| | Menstrual abnormalities |
| | Hirsutism |
| | Skin tags |
| | Sleep apnea |
| | Hypertension |
| | Diabetes |
| | Carpal tunnel |

**Clinical Pearls and Pitfalls**

- Galactorrhea was the presenting sign and prolactin was high which made the diagnosis initially seem to be a prolactinoma. However, in such patients with hyperprolactinemia and adenoma, particularly with any signs or symptoms of acromegaly, tests for GH excess should be obtained given that there can be co-secretion of prolactin and GH.

- When IGF-1 and GH show discrepant values, reasons for false positive and false negatives should be reviewed, and levels should be repeated in a reliable assay. If either value is confirmed, levels should be interpreted based on the clinical correlation and treated if there are symptoms or signs of acromegaly.

- Repeat surgery can be considered if remnant tumor is surgically accessible.

- Classic acromegaly appearance may not be obvious in early disease; enlargement of hands and feet may be only sign without facial features of acromegaly in some patients.

- Galactorrhea may be a sign of acromegaly in women.

- When acromegaly persists after surgery, medications should be administered to control GH and IGF-1 and tumor remnant; if a medication is ineffective alone, medical therapies can be combined.

- If medical therapy is not effective, not tolerated, or inaccessible, radiotherapy should be considered in patients in whom surgery has been unsuccessful.

- Following radiotherapy to the pituitary, long-term follow-up of anterior pituitary function should be evaluated at 6 months, 12 months, and yearly after the radiation therapy is completed since hormonal loss can occur for many years or even up to decades after the radiation therapy.

- This case was notable in that the original IGF-I was normal at diagnosis when she had isolated elevation of growth hormone; over time, as the disease progressed off therapy, her IGF-I level became elevated.

sweating, and subtle progression in facial features of acromegaly (Table 6.1). She was then treated with pegvisomant with normal IGF-1 levels. Annual MRI of the pituitary post-radiation demonstrated stability of the tumor. Anterior pituitary function tests were obtained at 6 and 12 months and yearly following radiation, and all remained normal except for the finding of central hypothyroidism 5 years after radiation.

# References

1. Melmed S. Acromegaly. N Engl J Med. 2006;355:2558–73.
2. Freda PU. Monitoring of acromegaly: what should be performed when GH and IGF-1 levels are discrepant? Clin Endocrinol (Oxf). 2009;71:166–70.
3. Frystyk J, Freda P, Clemmons DR. The current status of IGF-I assays—a 2009 update. Growth Horm IGF Res. 2010;20:8–18.
4. Freda PU. Current concepts in the biochemical assessment of the patient with acromegaly. Growth Horm IGF Res. 2003;13:171–84.
5. Cazabat L, et al. Germline inactivating mutations of the aryl hydrocarbon receptor-interacting protein gene in a large cohort of sporadic acromegaly: mutations are found in a subset of young patients with macroadenomas. Eur J Endocrinol. 2007;157:1–8.
6. Katznelson L, et al. Acromegaly: an Endocrine Society Clinical Practice Guideline. J Clin Endocrinol Metab. 2014;99:3933–51.
7. Fleseriu M, et al. Hormonal replacement in hypopituitarism in adults: an Endocrine Society Clinical Practice Guideline. J Clin Endocrinol Metab. 2016;101:3888–921.
8. Dineen R, Stewart PM, Sherlock M. Acromegaly. QJM. 2017;110(7):411–20. pii: hcw00.
9. Abs R, et al. Cabergoline in the treatment of acromegaly: a study in 64 patients. J Clin Endocrinol Metab. 1998;83:374–8.
10. Chang SC, Chen CH, Lu ML. Cabergoline-induced psychotic exacerbation in schizophrenic patients. Gen Hosp Psychiatry. 2008;30:378–80.
11. Barake M, et al. Investigation of impulsivity in patients on dopamine agonist therapy for hyperprolactinemia: a pilot study. Pituitary. 2014;17:150–6.
12. Shih HA, Loeffler JS. Radiation therapy in acromegaly. Rev Endocr Metab Disord. 2008;9:59–65.

# Chapter 7
# Acromegaly and Diabetes Mellitus: Special Considerations

Lindsay Fourman and Lisa B. Nachtigall

## Case Presentation

A 49-year-old man with a history of bipolar disorder, diabetes mellitus type 2 (DM2), hypertension, and hyperlipidemia presented to the hospital with psychosis and profound functional decline. The endocrinology team was consulted when he was noted to have random blood glucose of 526 mg/dL and 2+ urine ketones.

The patient reported a 10-year history of DM2 without any known complications. His blood glucose had been poorly controlled in recent months due to medication nonadherence in the setting of his psychiatric illness with an outpatient hemoglobin A1c (HbA1c) > 14%. He also reported the gradual worsening of his glycemic control over several years despite uptitration of antihyperglycemic agents by his primary care physician. His medication regimen at the time of admission was metformin, pioglitazone, canagliflozin, and dulaglutide. Family history was notable for a mother with DM2 but no other endocrine diseases.

On exam, his body mass index (BMI) was 30.2 kg/m² with blood pressure 134/87 mm Hg and pulse 94 beats per minute. The patient was noted to have frontal bossing, mandibular prognathism, macroglossia,

L. Fourman · L. B. Nachtigall (✉)
Neuroendocrine Unit, Massachusetts General Hospital,
Harvard Medical School, Boston, MA, USA
e-mail: lnachtigall@partners.org

© Springer International Publishing AG, part of Springer Nature 2018
L. B. Nachtigall (ed.), *Pituitary Tumors*,
https://doi.org/10.1007/978-3-319-90909-7_7

soft tissue swelling of the hands, and acanthosis nigricans of the posterior neck. Upon further questioning, he indicated that he had noted coarsening of his facial features, enlargement of his hands and feet, headaches, and increased diaphoresis over at least 10 years. However, he interpreted these signs and symptoms of acromegaly in the context of his psychiatric illness, believing that they were manifestations of a "curse" that had been placed upon him by his wife's family.

Given the patient's poor glycemic control with impaired insulin secretion as evidenced by 2+ urine ketones, he was started on a combination of short- and long-acting insulin that was increased to 100 units per day. Metformin was continued, but the patient's other antihyperglycemic agents were stopped to avoid polypharmacy. Serum insulin-like growth factor 1 (IGF-1) was 620 ng/mL (normal, 52–328 ng/mL), which was 3.7 standard deviations above his age- and sex-adjusted mean. All other hormonal axes were within normal limits. Pituitary magnetic resonance imaging (MRI) showed a 3 cm sellar and suprasellar mass consistent with a pituitary macroadenoma that displaced the optic chiasm and invaded the right cavernous sinus. Diffuse calvarial thickening also was noted. Formal visual field testing demonstrated bitemporal hemianopsia.

## My Management

(a) Transsphenoidal surgery by an experienced pituitary surgeon was recommended in order to debulk tumor in the setting of optic chiasm displacement.

(b) Postoperatively, blood glucose was closely monitored with insulin dose reductions made accordingly.

(c) A first-generation long-acting somatostatin analog (octreotide LAR) was recommended in order to control residual tumor postoperatively.

(d) Blood glucose was closely observed in the context of octreotide therapy initiation as levels may rise or fall.

## Assessment and Diagnosis

DM2 is a complication of acromegaly that is associated with an increased risk of cardiac disease [1] and mortality [2]. Concurrent diabetes also poses unique considerations for clinicians in terms of diagnosis and management of acromegaly.

The reported prevalence of DM2 in acromegaly has been highly variable with estimates ranging from 16 to over 50% [3, 4]. Patients with acromegaly have been shown to be at a higher risk of DM2 than the general population or non-acromegalic individuals with traditional diabetes risk factors [3, 5]. Increased BMI [5, 6], older age [5, 6], and family history of DM2 [6] all have been associated with impaired glucose tolerance in acromegaly, as in the general population. Longer pituitary disease duration [5] and higher IGF-1 (rather than GH) [6, 7] also predict disturbances in glucose homeostasis. In our patient, hyperglycemia may have been an early manifestation of GH excess since the onset of his DM2 dates back to when his acromegaly symptoms began. Additionally, the gradual rise in IGF-1 as his tumor grew over time may have accounted for the progressive deterioration of his glycemic control in recent years. His susceptibility to DM2 was likely further enhanced by his personal history of obesity (BMI 30.2 kg/m$^2$) and his family history of DM2. Notably, the endocrine consult team had been called to manage hyperglycemia, which led to the evaluation for acromegaly. Acromegaly should be considered in the differential diagnosis of disturbed glucose homeostasis and has been discovered incidentally in 0.6% of hospitalized patients with DM2 [8].

GH excess in acromegaly leads to DM2 by creating a state of insulin resistance. In a study using hyperinsulinemic-euglycemic clamp, acromegalic patients were shown to have defects in both hepatic and extrahepatic insulin action [9]. Extending these findings, GH was later shown to antagonize downstream mediators of insulin signaling including phosphoinositide (PI) 3-kinase [10]. GH also indirectly impairs insulin action by bringing about a rise in free fatty acids through the stimulation of lipolysis [11]. While insulin resistance is the primary disturbance in acromegaly, hyperglycemia only develops when pancreatic β cells can no longer keep up with the increased demand to secrete insulin. Several studies have shown that insulin resistance is similar among acromegalic patients irrespective of DM2 status, whereas a decline in β cell function was a distinguishing feature among individuals with prediabetes and diabetes [6, 12]. At the time of his hospital presentation, our patient had evidence of impaired β-cell function as evidenced by positive urine ketones although formal testing of insulin secretion (e.g., C-peptide) had not been obtained.

While IGF-1 is the preferred screening test for acromegaly [13], cases of acromegaly in the setting of poorly controlled DM2 have been described in which IGF-1 was falsely within the normal range. In these patients, IGF-1 subsequently rose to an abnormal value only once glycemic control was achieved with insulin therapy [14, 15]. For patients in whom IGF-1 is equivocal, GH suppression with oral glucose tolerance testing (OGTT) may be assessed [13]. However, an oral glucose load in diabetic individuals may fail to cause normal GH suppression such that false-positive results may occur [13, 16]. An OGTT also may be contraindicated for safety reasons among individuals with chronic hyperglycemia [17], and there is insufficient data to support the reliability of the OGTT to suppress GH while on insulin. Despite these considerations, our patient had a clearly elevated IGF-1, prompting his pituitary MRI without the need for further hormonal testing.

## Management

Acromegalic patients with comorbid DM2 often experience improved glycemic control following treatment of GH excess. Transsphenoidal surgery by an experienced surgeon is the treatment of choice in acromegaly for macroadenomas with local mass effect [13]. In one longitudinal study, 51% of acromegalic patients with baseline impaired glucose tolerance or DM2 experienced normalization of glucose homeostasis following surgical cure. In this study, individuals whose blood glucose derangements persisted had the most impaired β-cell function preoperatively [18]. Given the rapid decline in GH levels with surgery, close monitoring of blood glucose is required to avoid hypoglycemia, particularly in those receiving insulin or antihyperglycemic agents that may require dose adjustment.

While polyuria following resection of a pituitary adenoma commonly is attributed to diabetes insipidus (DI) [19], the differential diagnosis for postoperative diuresis in a diabetic acromegalic patient is broad. Resolution of soft tissue edema (i.e., diuresis of third-space fluid) is common following surgical control of acromegaly; a negative fluid balance on postoperative day 2 is predictive of a lower postoperative GH level [20]. Poor glycemic control due to surgical stress and/or the administration of intraoperative steroids also may result in polyuria. Thus, in acromegalic patients with comorbid DM2, concurrent sodium and glucose should be measured at regular intervals postoperatively, and signs/symptoms of DI besides polyuria should be assessed prior to the administration of desmopressin.

For patients in whom surgery is not appropriate or who have persistent disease despite surgical intervention, medical therapy with somatostatin analogs or the growth hormone receptor anatgonist is the treatment of choice [13]. The first generation somatostatin analogs (octreotide LAR and lanreotide) target somatostatin receptor subtype 2 and to a less extent receptor subtype 5 that are present in the pituitary and pancreas. Thus, though these agents may improve glucose homeostasis by reducing GH excess, they alternatively may exacerbate blood glucose levels by suppressing insulin secretion. Reassuringly, in a large meta-analysis of acromegalic patients, while fasting insulin decreased significantly with somatostatin analog treatment, marginal increases in fasting blood glucose and HbA1c were not significant. On the other hand, among the subset of patients with baseline DM2 or impaired glucose tolerance, glycemic control was noted to worsen in 25% of individuals [21].

Pasireotide is a second-generation somatostatin analog with affinity primarily for somatostatin receptor subtype 5 that may be used as an alternative to first-generation agents. In addition to inhibiting insulin secretion [22], pasireotide has been shown to reduce the secretion of glucagon-like peptide-1 (GLP-1) [23]. In a phase III clinical trial among medically naïve patients with acromegaly, long-acting pasireotide was associated with more hyperglycemic events (29% vs. 8%) and new diagnoses of DM2 (19% vs. 4%) compared to long-acting octreotide [24]. Another phase III study of pasireotide in acromegalic patients inadequately controlled on first-generation somatostatin analogs found that individuals with baseline DM2 or prediabetes were at increased risk of hyperglycemia-related adverse events compared to those with normal glucose tolerance [25]. Pegvisomant, a human GH receptor antagonist, has been shown to have more favorable effects on glucose homeostasis and may be an alternative for patients who develop progressive hyperglycemia in response to somatostatin analogs [13].

In acromegalic patients with comorbid DM2, glycemic control should be optimized prior to the initiation of somatostatin analog therapy, particularly in those who are high risk or who will receive pasireotide. Metformin has been recommended as the first-line agent to treat pasireotide-related hyperglycemia in patients with Cushing's disease [26]. A mechanistic study in healthy controls also has suggested that glucagon protein-1 (GLP-1) receptor agonists and dipeptidyl peptidase (DPP-4) inhibitors may be particularly efficacious to treat hyperglycemia on pasireotide, perhaps since these agents specifically target the GLP-1 pathway [22].

## Outcome

Our patient's elevated IGF-1 and macroadenoma on pituitary imaging were diagnostic of acromegaly. Given displacement of the optic chiasm, surgery was recommended as the first-line treatment option. However, in the context of the patient's recent psychiatric hospitalization, he was reluctant to undergo surgery and instead preferred medical therapy in the short term. Octreotide LAR 20 mg IM monthly was initiated. His blood glucoses were controlled prior to the initiation of therapy and were monitored following treatment initiation without a change in his insulin requirement.

One month after hospital discharge, the patient consented to and underwent transsphenoidal surgery with uncomplicated removal of sellar tumor. Residual tumor was noted in the right cavernous sinus on postoperative MRI. Pathology demonstrated pituitary adenoma that stained positive for GH with a Ki-67 proliferation rate of 0.5%. Somatostatin analog therapy was held for approximately two months following surgery to determine the bioactivity of residual disease at which time IGF-1 was 520 ng/mL (z-score 3.2). Accordingly, octreotide LAR was reinitiated at 30 mg IM monthly. Following three doses, IGF-1 partially downtrended to 407 ng/mL (z-score 2.5), and octreotide LAR was further uptitrated to 40 mg IM monthly. Three months later (7 months postoperatively), IGF-1 was 298 ng/mL (z-score 1.7), suggesting biochemical control on maximal octreotide therapy.

In the days following surgery, the patient experienced a noticeable diuresis with no hyperglycemia or change in serum sodium or thirst, consistent with mobilization of third-space fluid. The patient's blood glucose was monitored closely, and his insulin was downtitrated from 100 to 40 units daily within the first postoperative month. Following the reinitiation of octreotide, he experienced a marked reduction in headaches, diaphoresis, and soft tissue swelling that paralleled the biochemical improvement in his IGF-1. Insulin was further downtitrated and then discontinued while on maximum-dose octreotide, and DM2 subsequently was managed with metformin alone. With IGF-1 within the normal range, HbA1c was 6.9%.

In summary, control of GH excess in our patient corresponded to a remarkable reduction in his insulin resistance. Accordingly, despite the high dose of insulin that he needed preoperatively, insulin therapy was no longer required once biochemical control was achieved. As expected, our patient's DM2 did not resolve entirely with acromegaly treatment given that he had evidence of baseline β-cell dysfunction on initial presentation.

**Clinical Pearls and Pitfalls**
- DM2 is a common complication of acromegaly that is associated with heart disease and increased mortality.
- Acromegaly should be considered in the differential diagnosis of DM2, in the appropriate clinical context.
- Risk factors for impaired glucose tolerance in acromegaly include older age, increased BMI, family history of DM2, longer disease duration, and higher IGF-1.
- Poorly controlled DM2 may complicate the workup of acromegaly by leading to IGF-1 false negatives and OGTT false positives.

- Surgical or medical treatment of acromegaly may result in a reduction in insulin resistance such that decrease or discontinuation of antihyperglycemic agents may be appropriate.
- Somatostatin analogs, particularly pasireotide, may paradoxically worsen glycemic control despite improving GH excess.
- Postoperative polyuria in an acromegalic patient with comorbid DM2 may represent diabetes insipidus, diuresis of third-space fluids, or hyperglycemia.
- Pretreatment β-cell dysfunction predicts persistent abnormalities in glucose homeostasis despite acromegaly cure.

# References

1. Colao A, Baldelli R, Marzullo P, Ferretti E, Ferone D, Gargiulo P, et al. Systemic hypertension and impaired glucose tolerance are independently correlated to the severity of the acromegalic cardiomyopathy. J Clin Endocrinol Metab. 2000;85:193–9.
2. Rajasoorya C, Holdaway IM, Wrightson P, Scott DJ, Ibbertson HK. Determinants of clinical outcome and survival in acromegaly. Clin Endocrinol. 1994;41:95–102.
3. Dreval AV, Trigolosova IV, Misnikova IV, Kovalyova YA, Tishenina RS, Barsukov IA, et al. Prevalence of diabetes mellitus in patients with acromegaly. Endocr Connect. 2014;3:93–8.
4. Arosio M, Reimondo G, Malchiodi E, Berchialla P, Borraccino A, De Marinis L, et al. Predictors of morbidity and mortality in acromegaly: an Italian survey. Eur J Endocrinol. 2012;167:189–98.
5. Fieffe S, Morange I, Petrossians P, Chanson P, Rohmer V, Cortet C, et al. Diabetes in acromegaly, prevalence, risk factors, and evolution: data from the French Acromegaly Registry. Eur J Endocrinol. 2011;164:877–84.
6. Alexopoulou O, Bex M, Kamenicky P, Mvoula AB, Chanson P, Maiter D. Prevalence and risk factors of impaired glucose tolerance and diabetes mellitus at diagnosis of acromegaly: a study in 148 patients. Pituitary. 2014;17:81–9.
7. Niculescu D, Purice M, Coculescu M. Insulin-like growth factor-I correlates more closely than growth hormone with insulin resistance and glucose intolerance in patients with acromegaly. Pituitary. 2013;16:168–74.

8. Suda K, Fukuoka H, Iguchi G, Hirota Y, Nishizawa H, Bando H, et al. The prevalence of acromegaly in hospitalized patients with type 2 diabetes. Endocr J. 2015;62:53–9.
9. Hansen I, Tsalikian E, Beaufrere B, Gerich J, Haymond M, Rizza R. Insulin resistance in acromegaly: defects in both hepatic and extrahepatic insulin action. Am J Phys. 1986;250:E269–73.
10. del Rincon JP, Iida K, Gaylinn BD, McCurdy CE, Leitner JW, Barbour LA, et al. Growth hormone regulation of p85alpha expression and phosphoinositide 3-kinase activity in adipose tissue: mechanism for growth hormone-mediated insulin resistance. Diabetes. 2007;56:1638–46.
11. Higham CE, Rowles S, Russell-Jones D, Umpleby AM, Trainer PJ. Pegvisomant improves insulin sensitivity and reduces overnight free fatty acid concentrations in patients with acromegaly. J Clin Endocrinol Metab. 2009;94:2459–63.
12. Kasayama S, Otsuki M, Takagi M, Saito H, Sumitani S, Kouhara H, et al. Impaired beta-cell function in the presence of reduced insulin sensitivity determines glucose tolerance status in acromegalic patients. Clin Endocrinol. 2000;52:549–55.
13. Katznelson L, Atkinson JL, Cook DM, Ezzat SZ, Hamrahian AH, Miller KK, et al. American Association of Clinical Endocrinologists Medical guidelines for clinical practice for the diagnosis and treatment of acromegaly—2011 update: executive summary. Endocr Pract. 2011;17:636–46.
14. Lim DJ, Kwon HS, Cho JH, Kim SH, Choi YH, Yoon KH, et al. Acromegaly associated with type 2 diabetes showing normal IGF-1 levels under poorly controlled glycemia. Endocr J. 2007;54:537–41.
15. Wijayaratne DR, Arambewela MH, Dalugama C, Wijesundera D, Somasundaram N, Katulanda P. Acromegaly presenting with low insulin-like growth factor-1 levels and diabetes: a case report. J Med Case Rep. 2015;9:241.
16. Melmed S, Casanueva F, Cavagnini F, Chanson P, Frohman LA, Gaillard R, et al. Consensus statement: medical management of acromegaly. Eur J Endocrinol. 2005;153:737–40.
17. Rosario PW, Calsolari MR. Safety and specificity of the growth hormone suppression test in patients with diabetes. Endocrine. 2015;48:329–33.
18. Kinoshita Y, Fujii H, Takeshita A, Taguchi M, Miyakawa M, Oyama K, et al. Impaired glucose metabolism in Japanese patients with acromegaly is restored after successful pituitary surgery if pancreatic {beta}-cell function is preserved. Eur J Endocrinol. 2011;164:467–73.
19. Loh JA, Verbalis JG. Diabetes insipidus as a complication after pituitary surgery. Nat Clin Pract Endocrinol Metab. 2007;3:489–94.
20. Zada G, Sivakumar W, Fishback D, Singer PA, Weiss MH. Significance of postoperative fluid diuresis in patients undergoing transsphenoidal surgery for growth hormone-secreting pituitary adenomas. J Neurosurg. 2010;112:744–9.
21. Mazziotti G, Floriani I, Bonadonna S, Torri V, Chanson P, Giustina A. Effects of somatostatin analogs on glucose homeostasis: a metaanalysis of acromegaly studies. J Clin Endocrinol Metab. 2009;94:1500–8.

22. Breitschaft A, Hu K, Hermosillo Resendiz K, Darstein C, Golor G. Management of hyperglycemia associated with pasireotide (SOM230): healthy volunteer study. Diabetes Res Clin Pract. 2014;103:458–65.
23. Henry RR, Ciaraldi TP, Armstrong D, Burke P, Ligueros-Saylan M, Mudaliar S. Hyperglycemia associated with pasireotide: results from a mechanistic study in healthy volunteers. J Clin Endocrinol Metab. 2013;98:3446–53.
24. Colao A, Bronstein MD, Freda P, Gu F, Shen CC, Gadelha M, et al. Pasireotide versus octreotide in acromegaly: a head-to-head superiority study. J Clin Endocrinol Metab. 2014;99:791–9.
25. Gadelha MR, Bronstein MD, Brue T, Coculescu M, Fleseriu M, Guitelman M, et al. Pasireotide versus continued treatment with octreotide or lanreotide in patients with inadequately controlled acromegaly (PAOLA): a randomised, phase 3 trial. Lancet Diabetes Endocrinol. 2014;2:875–84.
26. Colao A, De Block C, Gaztambide MS, Kumar S, Seufert J, Casanueva FF. Managing hyperglycemia in patients with Cushing's disease treated with pasireotide: medical expert recommendations. Pituitary. 2014;17:180–6.

# Chapter 8
# Gigantism: Management of Fatigue and Daytime Sleepiness After Surgery and Radiation in Adolescents with GH Secreting Adenoma

**Vibha Singhal**

## Case Presentation

This is a 15-year-old girl who presents with coarse facial features and tall stature. History is negative for headaches, nausea, vision complaints, any obvious mucosal or skin lesions, or renal calculi. She uses continuous positive airway pressure (CPAP) at night and reports decreased exercise tolerance. Review of her growth charts reveals that her height percentiles started increasing at the age of 8 years (prepubertal). There is a family history of tall stature in maternal cousin who is 7 ft tall. Maternal grandmother died from "brain cancer," and further details could not be retrieved. Her midparental height is 5 ft 5 inches.

*Anthropometry*: Height: 191.3 cm (SD = +4.27); weight: 188 Lb (SD = +2.03); US/LS ratio = 1.06 (appropriate for age). Vitals were normal.

V. Singhal (✉)
Department of Pediatric Endocrinology, Massachusetts General Hospital, Harvard Medical School, Boston, MA, USA
e-mail: vsinghal1@partners.org

© Springer International Publishing AG, part of Springer Nature 2018    69
L. B. Nachtigall (ed.), *Pituitary Tumors*,
https://doi.org/10.1007/978-3-319-90909-7_8

*Pertinent exam findings*: Tall girl with coarse facial features who looked very different from her mother. There was no skin or mucosal findings. No organomegaly was noticed. No documented joint laxity. Visual field exam on confrontation was negative. She was Tanner 5 on breast examination (premenarchal).

*Biochemical testing*: TSH 1.20 mIU/mL (0.40–5.00), FreeT4 1.0 ng/dL (0.9–1.8). FSH 2.4 IU/L, LH 0.2 IU/L, EST <20 pg/mL, ACTH 25 pg/mL (6–76), CORT 4.2 mcg/dL, Prolactin 22.3 ng/dL (0.1–23.3), IGF-1846 ng/mL (218–659 for age and Tanner stage Z-SCORE 3.2), hemoglobin A1C 5.50.

OGTT had a nadir GH level of 35.9 ng/mL where normal OGTT nadir is <1 ng/mL. She passed her cosyntropin stimulation test.

*Imaging*: MRI revealed a sellar/suprasellar mass lesion measuring up to $39 \times 42 \times 44$ mm with bilateral cavernous sinus invasion. The optic chiasm was compressed and displaced along the anterosuperior aspect of the mass. There was encasement of the cavernous internal carotid arteries bilaterally.

Visual field testing was obtained which showed significant temporal defect in the left eye with good visual acuity and no afferent pupillary defect.

She was started on a somatostatin analog (SSA), lanreotide, to attempt tumor shrinkage for better surgical outcome. She was closely monitored for visual deterioration, and surgical resection was performed two months after the start of lanreotide treatment. She was also started on cabergoline at a dose of 0.5 mg weekly and oral contraceptives (OCPs). She subsequently developed central hypothyroidsm and secondary adrenal insufficiency and was placed on appropriate supplementation. She also received radiation for the residual tumor and continually elevated IGF-1 levels in the 700 s (218–659 ng/mL for age and Tanner stage). Her cabergoline dose was further increased to 0.5 mg every other day, and her IGF-1 entered the normal range at 378 ng/mL.

Over the course of next 6 months, she was noted to have increased rage, crying episodes, and the patient getting in trouble with teachers in school. She also developed extreme fatigue and sleepiness during the day and was awake at night. This was very debilitating and she was missing a lot of school. She had discontinued CPAP at night and was no longer snoring. She did not appear sad to her mother or her friends. She reported episodes where she would suddenly feel that she could not walk anymore and had to sit down instantly. Her IGF-1 level was normal at this point.

## My Management Options

(a) Discontinue cabergoline and request a sleep study
(b) Continue cabergoline and add pegvisomant
(c) Consider referral to a psychologist

## Assessment and Diagnosis

Excess growth hormone secretion before epiphyseal closure leads to gigantism. In most cases, it is a result of growth hormone excess from a pituitary tumor. The onset of symptoms at young age with the presence of family history warrants a genetic evaluation. The various syndromes associated with gigantism are listed in the Table 8.1.

As with most pituitary tumors, younger age at presentation is associated with more aggressive tumors [3]. Giant GH-secreting pituitary tumors are invasive and need a multimodal treatment approach to control GH excess and tumor growth [4]. Medical, surgical, and radiation therapy is often needed. Of note, much of the data comes from older patients with acromegaly and should be interpreted with that in mind.

*Medical therapy*: Somatostatin analogs (SSAs), dopamine ago-nists, and growth hormone receptor blockers are often used alone or in combination based on need and patient tolerability. SSA may also reduce the tumor size in about a third of patients [5, 6]. Dopamine agonists are usually used in conjunction with a SSA, and the combination may be effective in lowering the IGF-1 level further. Pegvisomant is a GH receptor antagonist and decreases the IGF-1 levels in a dose-dependent manner. As pegvisomant does not inhibit GH secretion, its use is associated with increase in

**Table 8.1** Syndromes associated with gigantism

| Syndrome | Gene | Associated features |
|---|---|---|
| Multiple endocrine neoplasia type 1 (MEN 1) | Menin (MEN 1) | Parathyroid, anterior pituitary, and pancreatic neuroendocrine tumors |
| Multiple endocrine neoplasia type 4 (MEN 4) [1] | Cyclin-dependent kinase inhibitor (CDKN1B) | Parathyroid, anterior pituitary, testicular, cervical, thyroid, adrenal, and renal tumors |
| Familial isolated pituitary adenoma (FIPA) | Aryl hydrocarbon receptor-interacting protein (AIP) | At least two members of the same family with pituitary tumor |
| McCune-Albright syndrome | GNAS1 encodes the alpha subunit of the stimulatory G protein (Gs) | Fibrous dysplasia, cafe-au-lait spots, precocious puberty |
| Carney complex | PPKAR1A | Skin pigmentation, cardiac myxomas, Cushing syndrome with pigmented nodular adrenocortical disease (PPNAD) |
| X-linked acrogigantism (X-LAG) | GPR101 encodes a G-protein coupled receptor | Median onset of gigantism is 12 months [2] |
| Paraganglioma, pheochromocytoma, and pituitary adenoma association (3PA) | Succinate dehydrogenase (SDH A-D) | Most cases are familial |

serum GH concentration. It may presumably lead to increase in adenoma size and initial radiological monitoring should be considered [7].

*Surgical therapy*: It is the treatment of choice for small and large tumors which are resectable and those which pose a risk to visual loss. The cure rate depends on the size of the tumor and the expertise of the surgeon.

*Radiation therapy*: It is recommended when there is residual tumor after surgery as it leads to decrease in tumor size and reduces IGF-1 concentrations in majority of the patients. It usually takes a few years to take effect and hence is used in situations where surgery and medical therapy are not effective.

There are many causes of extreme fatigue, daytime sleepiness, and mood changes in a patient with gigantism post TSS and radiation with panhypopituitarism.

**Disease Related**

1. Excess Growth Hormone: Fatigue is a commonly present at initial diagnosis and may persist with elevated GH and IGF-1 levels.
2. Adrenal Insufficiency: Adrenal insufficiency (AI) can present as fatigue. Cortisol levels (at 8am or stimulated) should be regularly monitored in patients with pituitary macroadenomas and/or radiation therapy as AI can develop years after radiation.
3. Hypogonadism: Hypogonadism may be associated with fatigue. Adequate replacement of gonadal steroids is important which also provides the additional benefit of lowering IGF-1 levels with exogenous estrogen in females.
4. Growth Hormone Deficiency: This can develop after surgery and radiation. It affects quality of life and is associated with decreased energy levels [8]. In a randomized controlled trial, growth hormone replacement in cured acromegaly patients led to improvement in quality of life [9].
5. Myopathy: There are reports of severe muscle tenderness in acromegaly which is associated with elevated creatinine kinase (CK-MB) levels. This should be considered and addressed with appropriate physical therapy.
6. Sleep Apnea: It is a recognized complication of acromegaly. Almost half of the patients with acromegaly suffer from sleep apnea. It is usually of obstructive nature resulting from soft tissue enlargement. Rarely, central sleep apnea from altered respiratory control is also reported and should be treated accordingly.
7. Narcolepsy is a neurological disorder characterized by irresistible sleep, sleep paralysis (momentary inability to move the body), and cataplexy (sudden transient loss of muscle tone—usually in response to an emotional trigger). The diagnosis is established by nocturnal polysomnography (PSG) and multiple sleep latency test (MSLT). It can be rarely seen in patients with brain

tumors and is reported in one case of acromegaly after radiation treatment [10]. Testing levels of hypocretin in CSF can be undertaken if the diagnosis of narcolepsy is equivocal. Pharmacotherapy with stimulants is usually the first line of treatment.

8. Respiratory Disorders: Mortality from respiratory disorders is threefold more common in acromegaly patients than in the general population [11]. Upper respiratory obstruction from macroglossia, mucosal, and tonsillar hypertrophy is common although pulmonary dysfunction and disturbance in central nervous system may occur. Involvement of lung parenchyma (decrease carbon monoxide diffusion capacity) has been shown before any detectable structural deficits appear in MRI [12].

9. Depression: Patients with acromegaly suffer from depression even long after medical cure [13]. This affects their overall quality of life, and some may develop somatic symptoms of fatigue and insomnia. This is an important consideration in evaluation of fatigue after acromegaly treatment.

**Treatment Related**

1. Radiation fatigue: Fatigue is a common acute and chronic complication of cranial radiation. In rare cases, radiation can cause "somnolence syndrome." It is more commonly seen in children than adults and usually occurs in the first 6 months after radiation [14]. This is associated with extreme sleepiness and maybe associated with symptoms of increased intracranial pressure. It is usually self-resolving.

2. Somatostatin analogs (SSAs): Quality of life may be impaired in acromegaly patients post-surgery if they need somatostatin analogs despite similar IGF-1 levels [15]. SSA usage in the long term was not, however, associated with declining self reported QOL [16].

3. Dopamine agonists (Cabergoline): Cabergoline is the more commonly used DA due to its better efficacy and safety profile. However, its use has been shown to be associated with fatigue, somnolence, impulsivity, and rage episodes. Most of these effects are dose dependent and reversible once the medication is discontinued [17].

## Psychosocial

Other factors like social conditions, recent changes in school, job, or parental discord should not be neglected and appropriately addressed.

# Management

### Evaluations

- The patient had an ACTH stimulation test to rule out adrenal insufficiency.
- She was referred to sleep specialist where she had sleep study and a multiple sleep latency test.
- She was seen by a psychologist to rule out mood disorder.

### Medication Changes

- Cabergoline was discontinued.
- Appropriate thyroid and estrogen replacement was continued.
- Pegvisomant was added at further follow-up as her IGF-1 was above normal range.

# Outcome

Her peak cortisol level on ACTH stimulation test was 14 mcg/dL, and we started her on low-dose steroid replacement. Patient was diagnosed with narcolepsy as she had significantly abnormal MSLT—multiple sleep latency test. She was started on modafinil—a stimulant. Patient developed anorexia with modafinil (known side effect) and lost weight. With close observation, she regained her appetite and the weight stabilized. Cabergoline was discontinued to see if her "aggressive" symptoms would improve. Over the next few weeks, aggressive symptoms were significantly improved. However, this led to an increase in her IGF-1 levels, and hence pegvisomant was added.

**Clinical Pearls and Pitfalls**
- Narcolepsy, albeit rare, can be a debilitating consequence of gigantism/acromegaly and its treatment. It should be diagnosed and managed by a sleep specialist. Patients are not allowed to drive unless their symptoms resolve substantially.
- Recognize that the side effect profile of medications may vary in adolescents as compared with adults. Cabergoline may cause "aggressiveness" in some teenagers.
- Close follow-up and monitoring of gigantism/acromegaly patients are important.

# References

1. Thakker RV. Multiple endocrine neoplasia type 1 (MEN1) and type 4 (MEN4). Mol Cell Endocrinol. 2014;386(1–2):2–15. https://doi.org/10.1016/j.mce.2013.08.002.
2. Trivellin G, Daly AF, Faucz FR, Yuan B, Rostomyan L, Larco DO, et al. Gigantism and acromegaly due to Xq26 microduplications and GPR101 mutation. N Engl J Med. 2014;371(25):2363–74. https://doi.org/10.1056/NEJMoa1408028.
3. Cazabat L, Libe R, Perlemoine K, Rene-Corail F, Burnichon N, Gimenez-Roqueplo AP, et al. Germline inactivating mutations of the aryl hydrocarbon receptor-interacting protein gene in a large cohort of sporadic acromegaly: mutations are found in a subset of young patients with macroadenomas. Eur J Endocrinol. 2007;157(1):1–8. https://doi.org/10.1530/EJE-07-0181.
4. Shimon I, Jallad RS, Fleseriu M, Yedinak CG, Greenman Y, Bronstein MD. Giant GH-secreting pituitary adenomas: management of rare and aggressive pituitary tumors. Eur J Endocrinol. 2015;172(6):707–13. https://doi.org/10.1530/EJE-14-1117.
5. Thapar K, Kovacs KT, Stefaneanu L, Scheithauer BW, Horvath E, Lloyd RV, et al. Antiproliferative effect of the somatostatin analogue octreotide on growth hormone-producing pituitary tumors: results of a multicenter randomized trial. Mayo Clin Proc. 1997;72(10):893–900. https://doi.org/10.1016/S0025-6196(11)63358-2.
6. Freda PU. Somatostatin analogs in acromegaly. J Clin Endocrinol Metab. 2002;87(7):3013–8. https://doi.org/10.1210/jcem.87.7.8665.

7. Buhk JH, Jung S, Psychogios MN, Goricke S, Hartz S, Schulz-Heise S, et al. Tumor volume of growth hormone-secreting pituitary adenomas during treatment with pegvisomant: a prospective multicenter study. J Clin Endocrinol Metab. 2010;95(2):552–8. https://doi.org/10.1210/jc.2009-1239.

8. Rosen T, Wiren L, Wilhelmsen L, Wiklund I, Bengtsson BA. Decreased psychological well-being in adult patients with growth hormone deficiency. Clin Endocrinol. 1994;40(1):111–6.

9. Miller KK, Wexler T, Fazeli P, Gunnell L, Graham GJ, Beauregard C, et al. Growth hormone deficiency after treatment of acromegaly: a randomized, placebo-controlled study of growth hormone replacement. J Clin Endocrinol Metab. 2010;95(2):567–77. https://doi.org/10.1210/jc.2009-1611.

10. Dempsey OJ, McGeoch P, de Silva RN, Douglas NJ. Acquired narcolepsy in an acromegalic patient who underwent pituitary irradiation. Neurology. 2003;61(4):537–40.

11. Murrant NJ, Gatland DJ. Respiratory problems in acromegaly. J Laryngol Otol. 1990;104(1):52–5.

12. Benfante A, Ciresi A, Bellia M, Cannizzaro F, Bellia V, Giordano C, et al. Early lung function abnormalities in acromegaly. Lung. 2015;193(3):393–9. https://doi.org/10.1007/s00408-015-9710-1.

13. Tiemensma J, Biermasz NR, van der Mast RC, Wassenaar MJ, Middelkoop HA, Pereira AM, et al. Increased psychopathology and maladaptive personality traits, but normal cognitive functioning, in patients after long-term cure of acromegaly. J Clin Endocrinol Metab. 2010;95(12):E392–402. https://doi.org/10.1210/jc.2010-1253.

14. Ryan J. Radiation somnolence syndrome. J Pediatr Oncol Nurs. 2000;17(1):50–3.

15. Postma MR, Netea-Maier RT, van den Berg G, Homan J, Sluiter WJ, Wagenmakers MA, et al. Quality of life is impaired in association with the need for prolonged postoperative therapy by somatostatin analogs in patients with acromegaly. Eur J Endocrinol. 2012;166(4):585–92. https://doi.org/10.1530/EJE-11-0853.

16. Khairi S, Sagvand BT, Pulaski-Liebert K, Tritos NA, Klibanski A, Nachtigall LB. Clinical Outcomes and Self-Reported Symptoms in patients with Acromegaly: An 8-Year Follow-up of a Lanreotide Study. Endocr Pract. 2017;23:56–65.

17. Webster J, Piscitelli G, Polli A, D'Alberton A, Falsetti L, Ferrari C, et al. The efficacy and tolerability of long-term cabergoline therapy in hyperprolactinaemic disorders: an open, uncontrolled, multicentre study. European Multicentre Cabergoline Study Group. Clin Endocrinol. 1993;39(3):323–9.

# Chapter 9
# A Rare Entity: TSH-Secreting Adenoma

Laura E. Dichtel

## Case Presentation

A 72-year-old male with past medical history of benign prostatic hypertrophy and migraines was found to have an elevated TSH of 5.2 μIU/mL (normal 0.356–3.740 μIU/mL) on routine screening. He denied any symptoms of hypothyroidism, including weight gain, fatigue, cold intolerance, constipation, or dry skin. TSH was rechecked and found to be 5.92 μIU/mL (normal 0.356–3.740 μIU/mL) with an elevated free T4 (FT4) of 2.14 ng/dL (normal 0.75–1.69 ng/dL). Despite the elevation in FT4, he was started on levothyroxine 75 mcg daily, which he took inconsistently for approximately one month only. TFTs repeated off of levothyroxine confirmed an elevated TSH of 6.08 μIU/mL (normal 0.356–3.740 μIU/mL) and concurrently elevated FT4 of 1.85 ng/dL (normal 0.76–1.46 ng/dL). Because of persistently abnormal thyroid function tests, he was referred to an endocrinologist. Full thyroid testing panel then revealed a TSH of 6.35 μIU/mL (normal 0.356–3.740 μIU/mL), total T4 of 13.5 μg/dL (normal 4.5–12.1 μg/dL), FT4 of 1.57 ng/dL (normal 0.76–1.46 ng/dL), and FT3 of 4.1 pg/mL (normal 2.0–3.5 pg/mL).

L. E. Dichtel (✉)
Neuroendocrine Unit, Massachusetts General Hospital,
Harvard Medical School, Boston, MA, USA
e-mail: ldichtel@partners.org

© Springer International Publishing AG, part of Springer Nature 2018     79
L. B. Nachtigall (ed.), *Pituitary Tumors*,
https://doi.org/10.1007/978-3-319-90909-7_9

## My Management

(a) Complete diagnostic workup to rule out other causes of central hyperthyroidism.
(b) Perform MRI to confirm the presence of a pituitary lesion.
(c) Once TSH-secreting pituitary adenoma is confirmed, discuss therapeutic options with the patient, including surgery, medical management with somatostatin analogs, and/or radiation.

## Epidemiology

Thyrotropinomas, or TSH-secreting adenomas are rare, estimated to comprise only 0.5–3% of pituitary tumors overall [1, 2]. They can be seen across the age spectrum, with reports of cases from age 8–84 years [3, 4] and a peak incidence between the fifth and seventh decade of life [2, 5]. Most studies report an equal prevalence between genders [6, 7], although a few series have noted a higher frequency in women (60–65%) as compared to men [2, 5]. TSH-secreting adenomas are predominantly benign, with only a few case reports of malignant transformation reported [8–11]. The majority are macroadenomas at the time of diagnosis (range 57–100% across one comprehensive review), with tumor invasion occurring in 23–91% of cases [3]. Published series report a hormonal co-secretion rate of up to 40%, mainly involving concurrent GH or prolactin overproduction [2, 3].

The majority of patients with TSH-secreting adenomas present with classic symptoms of hyperthyroidism, and, depending on the series, up to 70% have a history of misdiagnosed primary thyroid disease with either prior thyroidectomy and/or radioactive iodine treatment [3, 4, 12]. Up to 90% are reported to have a coexisting nonautonomous goiter, mainly due to TSH-stimulation over time [4]. Patients can alternatively come to medical attention due to classic symptoms of a pituitary macroadenoma, such as headache, visual field changes or symptoms of coexisting hypopituitarism, or a combination of mass effect-related symptoms in addition to hyperthyroidism [1, 4, 13]. Multiple authors have suggested that increased sensitivity of laboratory testing and incidental findings on head imaging have led to a change in the classic presentation of TSH-secreting adenomas over time, with more individuals presenting at earlier stages of biochemical disease and with smaller lesions than what is reflected in most historical series [3, 4, 7, 14].

## Diagnosis

The diagnosis of a TSH-secreting adenoma should be considered in the presence of an inappropriately normal to elevated TSH in conjunction with increased free serum thyroid hormone levels (FT4, FT3), which is termed central hyperthyroidism. However, the differential diagnosis of central hyperthyroidism includes a broad array of conditions that must first be exonerated [1]. Laboratory interference, for example, by heterophilic antibodies to mouse immunoglobulins, biotin supplementation (by interference with biotinylated laboratory assays), or concurrent use of heparin (which displaces T4 and T3 from TBG), can cause a biochemical picture of central hyperthyroidism in the absence of clinical symptoms [15]. These should be excluded through appropriate testing and review of all medication and over-the-counter supplement history. Central hyperthyroidism can also occur in other conditions, such as resistance to thyroid hormone (RTH) [16, 17], very early destructive thyroiditis, erratic compliance with thyroid hormone replacement, recent initiation of amiodarone, or due to laboratory interference in familial dysalbuminemic hyperthyroxinemia [18].

It is particularly important to rule out thyroid hormone resistance in patients with central hyperthyroidism, with RTHß being the most common form of thyroid hormone resistance. Patients with RTHß can have variable degrees of hormone resistance based on distribution of receptor subtypes but generally do not experience frank symptoms of hyperthyroidism. If any are present, the most commonly reported symptoms in RTHß include isolated goiter, hyperactivity, and/or tachycardia [16]. This is in contrast to patients with TSH-secreting adenomas, who generally experience a more significant and classic constellation of hyperthyroid symptoms [1]. Given that RTHß is most commonly inherited in a dominant fashion, family history of RTHß or biochemical screening of additional members can be helpful in confirming this diagnosis. Patients with TSH-secreting adenomas are more likely to present with a history of additional pituitary hormone abnormalities or symptoms due to mass effect from the lesion. Furthermore, SHBG tends to be elevated in TSH-secreting adenomas and normal in RTHß [19]. Finally, serum α-subunit can also be used to distinguish between RTHß and a likely TSH-secreting adenoma. Elevation in α-subunit as well as an α-subunit/TSH ratio > 1 [calculated as (α-subunit in ng/mL/TSH in μIU/mL) × 10] supports the diagnosis of TSH-secreting adenoma. However, the sensitivity and specificity of the α-subunit/TSH ratio has been called into question by multiple authors [1, 3], and this piece of data must be interpreted in the context of all available data and patient characteristics.

Dynamic testing can help differentiate TSH-secreting adenomas from RTHß and includes (1) TRH stimulation test, in which 90% of patients with TSH-secreting adenomas demonstrated a blunted response, and (2) T3 suppression test, in which the majority of patients with TSH-secreting adenomas lack the expected suppression of TSH. While some guidelines still recommend these dynamic tests [1], TRH is not available in the United States [20], and T3 administration should not be administered to older patients or those with certain coexisting conditions [3, 21]. Thus, the diagnosis of TSH-secreting adenoma in a patient with central hyperthyroidism is usually made based on clinical and family history, α-subunit testing, SHBG levels, pituitary MRI, and genetic testing for RTHß when appropriate.

In summary, once central hyperthyroidism is identified, a full workup should include evaluation for symptoms of hyperthyroidism, history of potentially confounding medications, measurement of heterophile antibodies, repeat thyroid function testing, and measurement of α-subunit and SHBG with consideration of the diagnosis of RTHß as discussed above. Pituitary MRI should be performed in patients who have not yet had radiographic evaluation. All patients with an identified pituitary lesion should undergo additional hormonal testing, including prolactin, IGF-1, morning cortisol, morning testosterone (men), and SHBG. Menstrual history should also be obtained as clinical assessment of gonadal function in women and estradiol and LH and FSH should be obtained in premenopausal women with absent or irregular menses. Patients who are found to have a macroadenoma should additionally undergo a standard 250 mcg cosyntropin stimulation test to prove adrenal sufficiency if morning cortisol is not found to be adequate ($\geq 18$ mcg/dL).

## Management

Therapeutic options for patients with TSH-secreting adenomas include transsphenoidal pituitary surgery, medical treatment with somatostatin analogs (SSAs), and radiation therapy. Transsphenoidal pituitary surgery is considered the first-line treatment for TSH-secreting adenomas [1]. Surgery can be considered definitive therapy in the case of complete resection, or as a debulking procedure when the former is not possible. However, there is a concern in the literature that surgical complications may be more prevalent in patients with TSH-secreting adenomas compared with other pituitary adenoma subtypes, possibly due to the fibrotic nature of TSH-secreting lesions [14]. A recent review of all surgical series from 1993 to 2014 demonstrated that, on average, 70% of surgical patients were euthyroid postoperatively and 62% demonstrated no residual tumor [3]. Recurrence rates of up to 31% postoperatively have been noted [22], and these patients should be followed closely even if initially thought to be in remission after surgery. However, the limitations of these surgical series include small numbers, heterogeneity of patient populations, and varying study methodologies. Thus, surgery remains the primary recommended treatment for TSH-secreting adenomas [1], but is often used in conjunction with medical management and/or radiotherapy.

Medical management has been found to be quite effective in patients with TSH-secreting adenomas [1, 23], which have been shown to express somatostatin receptors (particularly SSTR2 and SSTR5). Series report normalization of thyroid function tests in 90% of patients, with significant reduction in tumor size in 30–55% of patients [1, 3, 6, 24]. SSAs can be used for preoperative normalization of thyroid hormone levels (with or without methimazole), as primary medical treatment if surgery is contraindicated or declined, or for residual disease in postoperative patients. Patients on SSAs should be monitored for the development of hyperglycemia, gallbladder disease, and gastrointestinal side effects. Of note, dopamine agonists have also been utilized as medical therapy in TSH-secreting adenomas. However, they have only been found to induce biochemical control in a small subset of mixed prolactin/TSH-secreting tumors [7, 24].

Finally, radiation therapy can be used as definitive therapy in patients who do not have surgery or in patients with residual disease postoperatively who do not want to commit to long-term SSA treatment or in whom SSA treatment has failed. Postoperative series report that approximately 10–48% of patients have historically undergone subsequent radiation therapy. However, there is a significant risk of hypopituitarism with radiation therapy, as expected with radiation therapy for any pituitary tumor subtype.

In summary, TSH-secreting adenomas are rare but must be considered in the differential diagnosis of central hyperthyroidism. While historically TSH-secreting adenomas were more likely to present as macroadenomas, more recent series demonstrate a higher prevalence of microadenomas at diagnosis than previously reported, likely due to earlier detection. Treatment options include transsphenoidal surgery, medical therapy with SSAs, radiation, or some combination of the three. The goal of therapy involves both normalization of thyroid function, alleviation of mass effect when present, and long-term control of lesion size. As in this case, choice of treatment modality can be based on a combination of clinical characteristics and patient preference. Regardless of treatment, these patients should have long-term endocrine follow-up with continued biochemical and radiologic surveillance.

## Outcome

Thyroid receptor beta mutation testing was negative. Alpha-subunit was elevated at 1.14 ng/mL (normal 0.09–0.76 ng/mL) with a concurrent TSH of 5.98 µIU/mL (normal 0.4–5.0 µIU/mL), giving a ratio [(α-subunit/TSH × 10)] of 1.9 (normal <1). Heterophile antibody was checked and found to be negative. The patient was not taking any biotin-containing supplements. Upon further questioning, he denied symptoms of hyperthyroidism, including weight loss, tachycardia, palpitations, exercise intolerance, muscle weakness, shortness of breath, heat intolerance, hyperdefecation, or increased anxiety. He did note a newly present fine tremor. He denied any vision changes or headaches outside of his normal pattern of migraines. Libido was normal, and he was treated successfully with tadalafil for erectile dysfunction. His only other medication was tamsulosin for benign prostatic hypertrophy. He had no family history of hyperthyroidism or other known endocrine disorders. On physical exam, he was well-appearing with normal blood pressure and heart rate. He had no proptosis or lid lag. Visual fields were intact to confrontation. Thyroid was small (10 gm) but palpable. A fine tremor was noted bilaterally. Lower extremity patellar reflexes were brisk bilaterally. The remainder of his exam was normal.

The patient underwent an MRI, which showed a 0.9 × 0.6 × 0.6 cm hypodensity of the right aspect of the pituitary gland without any optic nerve or chiasm compression. Further workup was obtained, including a normal AM cortisol (>18), testosterone, and prolactin. IGF-1 was slightly elevated at 191 ng/mL (normal 42–187 ng/mL) but was repeated in a different assay and was normal at 199 ng/mL (34–245 ng/mL). Given consistent evidence of a likely TSH-secreting adenoma, the patient was referred to a neurosurgeon who specialized in transsphenoidal procedures. Surgery to remove the presumed pituitary adenoma was recommended due to hormone secretion and size. However, the patient wished to undergo the least invasive treatment possible. As there was no concern for imminent mass effect upon optic structures, he was treated with a monthly somatostatin injection (lanreotide 90 mg). Baseline liver function testing and HbA1c were in the normal range prior to initiation of treatment. He experienced diarrhea for two weeks after the first injection and for one day following the second injection, 30 days later. He otherwise tolerated the medication well and had no further gastrointestinal side effects.

Approximately 5 weeks after starting treatment, TFTs normalized to a TSH of 4.96 µIU/mL (normal 0.4–5.0 µIU/mL), total T4 8.7 µg/dL (normal 4.5–10.9 µg/dL), FT4 1.6 ng/dL (normal 0.9–1.8 ng/dL), T3 154 ng/dL (normal 60–181 ng/dL), α-subunit 0.5 ng/mL (normal <0.5 ng/mL), and α-subunit/TSH ratio of 1.0 (normal <1). His tremor had improved and was only intermittent. On physical exam, his reflexes were present but normal. Liver function testing and hemoglobin A1c (HbA1c) remained normal on treatment.

MRI was repeated after 1 year on treatment and revealed a stable to slightly decreased 0.8 × 0.4 × 0.7 cm hypoenhancing lesion in the right pituitary gland with no mass effect. TFTs revealed a TSH of 2.43 µIU/mL (normal 0.45–5.0 µIU/mL), total T4 of 5.9 µg/dL (normal 4.5–10.9 µg/dL), FT4 of 1.0 ng/dL (normal 0.9–1.8 ng/dL), T3 78 ng/dL (normal 60-181 ng/dL), α-subunit of 0.4 ng/mL (normal <0.5 ng/mL), and α-subunit/TSH ratio of 1.6 (normal <1). The patient felt well with no complaints. Based on normalization of thyroid function testing, stability of the lesion, and his preference to minimize intervention, the lanreotide dosing interval was extended from 90 mg every 4 weeks to 90 mg every 6 weeks. TFTs on this dose remained in the normal range, with a TSH of 3.36 µIU/mL (normal 0.45–5.0 µIU/mL), FT4 1.1 ng/dL (normal 0.9–1.8 ng/dL), T3 92 ng/dL (normal 60–181 ng/dL), α-subunit of 0.3 ng/mL (normal <0.5 ng/mL), and α-subunit/TSH ratio of 0.9 (normal <1). MRI 2 years after starting treatment again showed a small reduction of the lesion size to 0.5 cm in diameter. He continues to defer surgical management and has tolerated SSA therapy well.

Given his age and history of hyperthyroidism, the patient underwent a bone density scan that revealed osteoporosis based on T scores of −1.6, −2.6, and −2.8 in the hip, spine, and forearm, respectively. Secondary osteoporosis workup was otherwise negative. He was started on alendronate, which he tolerated well. He continues to be followed closely in a neuroendocrine clinic with regular biochemical and radiologic surveillance.

**Clinical Pearls and Pitfalls**

- Central hyperthyroidism is defined as inappropriately normal to elevated TSH in conjunction with increased free serum thyroid hormone levels (FT4, FT3).
- Thyrotropinomas, or TSH-secreting adenomas, are rare; however, they must be considered in the differential diagnosis of central hyperthyroidism.
- While historically TSH-secreting adenomas were more likely to present as macroadenomas, more recent series demonstrate a higher prevalence of microadenomas at diagnosis than previously reported.
- Once a pituitary lesion has been identified, a full pituitary hormone workup should be completed. Neuro-ophthalmology evaluation is also required in the case of macroadenomas with concern for optic nerve or chiasm involvement.
- Therapeutic options for patients with TSH-secreting adenomas include transsphenoidal pituitary surgery, medical treatment with somatostatin analogs (SSAs), radiation therapy, or a combination of these modalities. The goals of therapy involve normalization of thyroid function, alleviation of mass effect when present, and long-term control of lesion size.
- While surgical treatment is still considered as the first-line, definitive therapy, the high efficacy of somatostatin analogs for the treatment of TSH-secreting adenomas provides another option for appropriate patients who prefer a non-surgical treatment plan.
- Regardless of treatment, these patients should have long-term endocrine follow-up with continued biochemical and radiologic surveillance.

# References

1. Beck-Peccoz P, Lania A, Beckers A, Chatterjee K, Wemeau JL. European thyroid association guidelines for the diagnosis and treatment of thyrotropin-secreting pituitary tumors. Eur Thyroid J. 2013;2:76–82.
2. Onnestam L, Berinder K, Burman P, et al. National incidence and prevalence of TSH-secreting pituitary adenomas in Sweden. J Clin Endocrinol Metab. 2013;98:626–35.
3. Amlashi FG, Tritos NA. Thyrotropin-secreting pituitary adenomas: epidemiology, diagnosis, and management. Endocrine. 2016;52:427–40.
4. Beck-Peccoz P, Persani L, Mannavola D, Campi I. Pituitary tumours: TSH-secreting adenomas. Best Pract Res Clin Endocrinol Metab. 2009;23:597–606.
5. Mindermann T, Wilson CB. Age-related and gender-related occurrence of pituitary adenomas. Clin Endocrinol. 1994;41:359–64.
6. Yamada S, Fukuhara N, Horiguchi K, et al. Clinicopathological characteristics and therapeutic outcomes in thyrotropin-secreting pituitary adenomas: a single-center study of 90 cases. J Neurosurg. 2014;121:1462–73.
7. Malchiodi E, Profka E, Ferrante E, et al. Thyrotropin-secreting pituitary adenomas: outcome of pituitary surgery and irradiation. J Clin Endocrinol Metab. 2014;99:2069–76.
8. Brown RL, Muzzafar T, Wollman R, Weiss RE. A pituitary carcinoma secreting TSH and prolactin: a non-secreting adenoma gone awry. Eur J Endocrinol. 2006;154:639–43.
9. Lee W, Cheung AS, Freilich R. TSH-secreting pituitary carcinoma with intrathecal drop metastases. Clin Endocrinol. 2012;76:604–6.
10. Nguyen HD, Galitz MS, Mai VQ, Clyde PW, Glister BC, Shakir MK. Management of coexisting thyrotropin/growth-hormone-secreting pituitary adenoma and papillary thyroid carcinoma: a therapeutic challenge. Thyroid. 2010;20:99–103.
11. Poggi M, Monti S, Pascucci C, Toscano V. A rare case of follicular thyroid carcinoma in a patient with thyrotropin-secreting pituitary adenoma. Am J Med Sci. 2009;337:462–5.
12. Brucker-Davis F, Oldfield EH, Skarulis MC, Doppman JL, Weintraub BD. Thyrotropin-secreting pituitary tumors: diagnostic criteria, thyroid hormone sensitivity, and treatment outcome in 25 patients followed at the National Institutes of Health. J Clin Endocrinol Metab. 1999;84:476–86.
13. Sanno N, Teramoto A, Osamura RY. Thyrotropin-secreting pituitary adenomas. Clinical and biological heterogeneity and current treatment. J Neuro-Oncol. 2001;54:179–86.
14. Socin HV, Chanson P, Delemer B, et al. The changing spectrum of TSH-secreting pituitary adenomas: diagnosis and management in 43 patients. Eur J Endocrinol. 2003;148:433–42.
15. Koulouri O, Moran C, Halsall D, Chatterjee K, Gurnell M. Pitfalls in the measurement and interpretation of thyroid function tests. Best Pract Res Clin Endocrinol Metab. 2013;27:745–62.

16. Beck-Peccoz P, Chatterjee VK. The variable clinical phenotype in thyroid hormone resistance syndrome. Thyroid. 1994;4:225–32.
17. Refetoff S, Weiss RE, Usala SJ. The syndromes of resistance to thyroid hormone. Endocr Rev. 1993;14:348–99.
18. Cartwright D, O'Shea P, Rajanayagam O, et al. Familial dysalbuminemic hyperthyroxinemia: a persistent diagnostic challenge. Clin Chem. 2009;55:1044–6.
19. Beck-Peccoz P, Brucker-Davis F, Persani L, Smallridge RC, Weintraub BD. Thyrotropin-secreting pituitary tumors. Endocr Rev. 1996;17:610–38.
20. Rapaport R, Akler G, Regelmann MO, Greig F. Time for thyrotropin releasing hormone to return to the United States of America. Thyroid. 2010;20:947–8.
21. Beck-Peccoz P, Persani L, Lania A. Thyrotropin-secreting pituitary adenomas. In: De Groot LJ, Chrousos G, Dungan K, et al., editors. Endotext. South Dartmouth, MA: MDText.com, Inc.; 2000.
22. Kirkman MA, Jaunmuktane Z, Brandner S, Khan AA, Powell M, Baldeweg SE. Active and silent thyroid-stimulating hormone-expressing pituitary adenomas: presenting symptoms, treatment, outcomes, and recurrence. World Neurosurg. 2014;82:1224–31.
23. van Varsseveld NC, Bisschop PH, Biermasz NR, Pereira AM, Fliers E, Drent ML. A long-term follow-up study of eighteen patients with thyrotrophin-secreting pituitary adenomas. Clin Endocrinol. 2014;80:395–402.
24. Beck-Peccoz P, Persani L. Medical management of thyrotropin-secreting pituitary adenomas. Pituitary. 2002;5:83–8.

# Index

© Springer International Publishing AG, part of Springer Nature 2018     91
L. B. Nachtigall (ed.), *Pituitary Tumors*,
https://doi.org/10.1007/978-3-319-90909-7

Printed in the United States
By Bookmasters